It Happened to Me

Series Editor: Arlene Hirschfelder

Books in the "It Happened to Me" series are designed for inquisitive teens digging for answers about certain illnesses, social issues, or lifestyle interests. Whether you are deep into your teen years or just entering them, these books are gold mines of up-to-date information, riveting teen views, and great visuals to help you figure out stuff. Besides special boxes highlighting singular facts, each book is enhanced with the latest reading list, web sites, and an index. Perfect for browsing, there's loads of expert information by acclaimed writers to help parents, guardians, and librarians understand teen illness, tough situations, and lifestyle choices.

1. *Learning Disabilities: The Ultimate Teen Guide,* by Penny Hutchins Paquette and Cheryl Gerson Tuttle, 2003.
2. *Epilepsy: The Ultimate Teen Guide,* by Kathlyn Gay and Sean McGarrahan, 2002.
3. *Stress Relief: The Ultimate Teen Guide,* by Mark Powell, 2002.
4. *Making Sexual Decisions: The Ultimate Teen Guide,* by L. Kris Gowen, Ph.D., 2003.
5. *Asthma: The Ultimate Teen Guide,* by Penny Hutchins Paquette, 2003.

Asthma

The Ultimate Teen Guide

PENNY HUTCHINS PAQUETTE

It Happened to Me, No. 5

The Scarecrow Press, Inc.
Lanham, Maryland • Toronto • Plymouth, UK

SCARECROW PRESS, INC.

Published in the United States of America
by Scarecrow Press, Inc.
A wholly owned subsidary of
The Rowman & Littlefield Publishing Group, Inc.
4501 Forbes Boulevard, Suite 200, Lanham, Maryland 20706
www.scarecrowpress.com

Estover Road
Plymouth PL6 7PY
United Kingdom

British Library Cataloguing in Publication Information Available

The hardback edition of this book was previously cataloged by the Library of Congress
as follows:

Paquette, Penny Hutchins.
    Asthma : the ultimate teen guide / Penny Hutchins Paquette.
        p. cm. — (It happened to me ; no. 5)
    Includes bibliographical references and index.
Contents: How long has this been going on? A history of asthma — What
is it? Asthma defined — Diagnosing asthma — Asthma triggers and how to
avoid them — What to do about it? Asthma treatments — Dealing with
asthma at school — When asthma becomes deadly — Coping with asthma —
On your own.
    ISBN 0-8108-4633-0
    1. Asthma—Juvenile literature. [1. Asthma. 2. Diseases.] I. Title.
II. Series.
RC591 .P355 2003
616.2'38—dc21   2002153542

ISBN: 0-8108-4633-0 (hardcover)
ISBN: 978-0-8108-5759-9 / 0-8108-5759-6 (paper)

♾™ The paper used in this publication meets the minimum requirements of
American National Standard for Information Sciences—Permanence of
Paper for Printed Library Materials, ANSI/NISO Z39.48-1992.
Manufactured in the United States of America.

For Bob

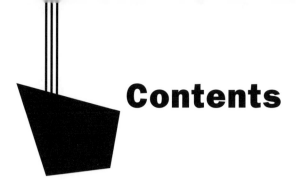

Contents

Acknowledgments

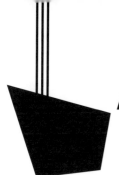

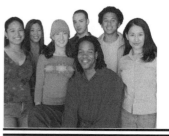

A special thanks to the young people who helped me remember what it is like to be a teenager with asthma, especially to Amit, Ashley, Alex, Michael, Torrey, Derek, Michele, Sam, Gillian, Chemise, and Katie. Thanks also to school nurses Mary Homan and Paula Dobrow for providing me with background information and for putting me in touch with young people who have asthma.

A debt of gratitude to allergy and asthma specialist Dr. Paul Hannaway for sharing his expertise and for his expert review of the manuscript.

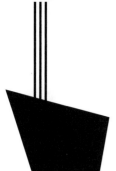

Introduction

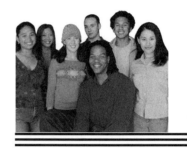

I had my first asthma attack more than 25 years ago. I was playing tennis. As I ran around the court, I began to cough. This wasn't the first time that had happened, but I assumed I had a cold and that the cough was a lingering one. This time, however, the cough was so violent that I had to stop playing and sit down. Even after I stopped, I had trouble catching my breath. It was a frightening experience and one that 17 million Americans can identify with today.

If you are a young person with asthma, perhaps you have had a similar experience. Maybe you find yourself short of breath when you exercise, or maybe you find you wheeze during certain times of the year. You could be among those who have allergies and find certain environmental factors trigger episodes. Maybe your asthma is mild and comes and goes infrequently, or maybe your asthma is more severe requiring daily medications and frequent monitoring. No matter what your symptoms are, and they vary greatly from person to person, if you are a teen with asthma, you are not alone. Today more than 4.8 million young people under eighteen have asthma. According to asthma researchers many asthmatic teenagers don't have enough information about the disease. That's especially unfortunate as information is one of the key ingredients for managing asthma.

I wrote this book to help improve that situation. It is not intended as a medical guide. I am not a doctor; I am a writer with asthma. *Asthma: The Ultimate Teen Guide* is just that, a guide. It will help guide you through the information that will help you better understand your condition. There is important information on the changes that happen in your body when you have an asthma attack, information about specific triggers that may make your asthma worse, an overview of medications that can help, and guidelines for monitoring your symptoms to help you know when your asthma may be getting worse.

There is also information from other young people just like you. Young men and women who are coping with asthma every day. They provide a *real person* point of view that may help you recognize that there are many out there coping with asthma, and they provide advice from a teen perspective. Some of these young people have mild asthma. Some have more serious symptoms, and some have faced life-threatening situations while learning to manage their disease. All of them understand what you are going through.

As you read *Asthma: The Ultimate Teen Guide* you will begin to gather the information you need to help you take on more of the responsibility of managing your asthma. If you are one of those young people who wants more control over his or her life, the information here will help you do just that. As you learn to monitor and record your symptoms and triggers, you will be able to give your doctor the information necessary to develop a plan that is right for you.

If you have just been diagnosed with asthma, this book will provide all the basic information you need to begin understanding asthma, the treatment of asthma, and how to cope with it. If you have had asthma for years and now want to begin taking an active part in working with your doctor, this book will help give you the confidence to discuss the disease with your doctor and with your parents. Whether your symptoms are mild or more serious, there is information here to help you become more independent.

So, read on, gather information, and start developing a plan of attack that will help you make the most of your life.

How Long Has This Been Going On? A History of Asthma

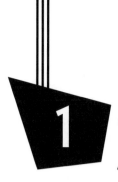

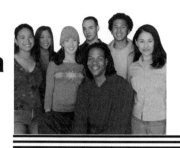

The first articles about asthma didn't appear in *The New York Times*, *The Boston Globe*, or *The Baltimore Sun*. In fact, descriptions of asthma were recorded long before any newspaper was in print. The ancient Egyptians were the first to produce a written description of asthma symptoms 5,000 years ago. The Ebers' Papyrus, the oldest preserved medical document, describes inhalation therapy for the treatment of asthma-like symptoms. Cardiologist and Egypt historian Dr. Sameh M. Arab provides this translation of the ancient treatment:

> *"You should then bring seven stones and heat them on fire. Take one of them, place parts of these drugs over it, cover it with a new jar with a pierced bottom. Introduce a tube of reed through this hole and put your mouth on this tube so that you swallow its fumes."*

The famous Greek physician Hippocrates, who was the first to use the word *asthma* to describe the illness, recommended purging and bleeding as treatment. The Romans were the first to understand that asthma was caused by an obstruction in the bronchial tubes, but they also thought a mixture of owl's blood and wine might provide a cure.

Chicken soup, a more appetizing choice, was first suggested as an asthma treatment by rabbi and physician Moses Maimonides in the 12th century. The Spanish rabbi, doctor, and philosopher was a pioneer in treating the whole patient with what we call holistic medicine today. After fleeing persecution from Cordova, Spain, he settled in Cairo and began practicing medicine. His success as a physician earned him an appointment to the Royal Court of Saladin,

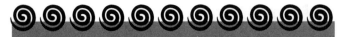

ANCIENT ASTHMATICS

Hippocrates (460–357 B.C.)

The word *asthma* comes from the Greek word *panos*, or panting. One of the first people to write about asthma was Hippocrates, who has been called "The Father of Medicine." Hippocrates believed that asthma was caused by moisture, occupation, and climate.

Lucius Annaeus Seneca (4 B.C.–79 A.D.)

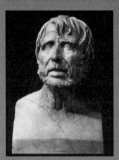

Seneca, a Roman statesman and writer remembered for his plays *The Trojan Women, Oedipus, Medea, The Mad Hercules, The Phoenician Women, Phaedra, Agamemnon,* and *Thyestes,* suffered from asthma. He compared his asthma episodes to a "last gasp" for air and said "nothing seems to me more troublesome." As a young man he was sent from Rome to Egypt in an attempt to help clear his asthma symptoms. Seneca tutored Nero, who would later become emperor of Rome.

Library of Congress photo, LC-US2-62-85059

Pliny the Elder (23–79 A.D.)

Roman scholar Pliny the Elder, best known for his scientific writings, suffered from chronic asthma. He is best remembered for his thirty-seven-volume encyclopedia, *Natural History.* Perhaps his asthma inspired him to study the medicinal qualities of herbs and other plants. When Mt. Vesuvius erupted in 79 A.D., he went to witness the eruption and suffocated from exposure to the sulfurous fumes.

Regent of Egypt. One of his specialties was the treatment of asthma. His *Treatise on Asthma* is still highly regarded today.

He believed those with asthma should be treated as individuals and that the focus should be on the treatment of the patient, not the disease. He recognized that eating well, exercising, maintaining a healthy weight, breathing clean air, and attending to personal hygiene were beneficial and that those treating patients should also recognize the importance of treating the spirit as well. Music, humor, stories, cheerful books, and visits from friends could provide a boost to the spirit.

ALLERGIES AND IRRITANTS SUSPECTED

Renaissance mathematician, inventor, and physician Girolamo Cardano is credited with curing John Hamilton, the Catholic Archbishop of Scotland, of asthma in the mid-1500s. Cardano, even then, recognized that a specific trigger might be causing asthma symptoms in the Archbishop. When the Archbishop switched from down-stuffed pillows and mattress to those stuffed with spun silk, his symptoms disappeared, and he declared himself cured.

In the 1600s, Konrad Schneider believed that dust and other irritants were responsible for the disease.

Personal experience helped Sir John Floyer understand asthma. His *A Treatise on Asthma* was published in 1698. As a physician and an asthma sufferer he recognized that the environment influenced his own symptoms. Although he never had asthma attacks while in Oxford, he often had a "fit or two" when visiting his home in Staffordshire. He observed that the smoky air affected his patients in London. He was among the first to recognize that asthma could be continuous or what he called *periodic convulsive asthma*. He developed his belief that asthma was caused by constrictions of the bronchi when he dissected a broken-winded horse.

DIAGNOSTIC INVENTIONS

Leopold Auenbrugger, an Austrian physician, used childhood activities as the basis for his scientific research. As a boy, he noticed he could determine how much wine was in a wine cask by tapping on the end of the barrel. As a physician, he began tapping on his patients' chests and noticed differences in the sounds created. He called his method *percussion* of the chest and used it to determine the amount of fluid in a patient's chest as well as the size of the patient's heart.

In the early 1800s, French physician René Laënnec discovered another method of determining what was happening inside his patients' bodies. He held a paper tube to a patient's chest and clearly heard the heartbeat. From his observations, he went on to invent the first stethoscope, which he made of wood. With this new instrument, doctors could hear the specific sounds associated with specific illnesses, including the wheezing sounds of asthma.

In the 1800s, French physician René Laënnec invented the first stethoscope.

Improvements in microscope technology further improved diagnostic procedures. By the 1830s, doctors could examine both lung tissue and lung secretions to help determine the cause of a patient's breathing problems.

Doctors began to better understand how air flowed into and out of the lungs with John Hutchinson's invention of the spirometer around 1850. With this new device, doctors could accurately measure what Hutchinson called vital capacity, the size of a maximum breath. This measurement could help doctors detect breathing difficulties before they would be heard with a stethoscope. Today's peak flow meters have their origins in this invention.

Although doctors could now hear breath sounds and measure breathing capacity, it wasn't until German physicist Wilhelm Roentgen invented the x-ray in 1895 that they could actually see what was happening inside the body. Roentgen didn't patent his invention, and before long, x-ray machines were being produced worldwide. The new technology was introduced in the United States in 1896.

INTEREST IN TRIGGERS RENEWED

At about the same time, English physician Henry Hyde Salter was gathering information about his patients' asthma and his own symptoms as well. His observations linked dust, cold air, and animal dander to asthmatic symptoms. He gathered his observations in his book, *On Asthma: Its Pathology and Treatment*. Like Moses Maimondes five hundred years earlier, Salter believed asthma patients had to be treated individually.

STRUGGLING TO BREATHE

The horrors of the asthmatic paroxysm far exceed any acute bodily pain: . . . The sense of impending suffocation, the agonizing struggle for the breath of life are so terrible they cannot be witnessed without sharing in the sufferer's distress. . . .
H. H. Salter

On Asthma: Its Pathology and Treatment.
2nd ed. London, England: Churchill; 1898.

DUSTY DISCUSSIONS

By the early 1920s, asthma research began to focus on the role of house dust as a trigger for asthma symptoms. R. A. Kern believed house dust was the primary cause of asthma. In the early 1920s, two brothers, S. S. Leopold and C. S. Leopold treated asthmatics by moving them to a dust-free room. A few years later, Willem Storm van Leeuwen suspected that dust mites (read more about this in chapter 4) in house dust might be provoking asthma symptoms. He, too, moved his patients from their homes to test the theory and created a specialized chamber to treat his patients.

The ancients started the process that helps us understand asthma, and researchers today continue to explore factors that trigger and treat the disorder. You can read more about that in the next chapters.

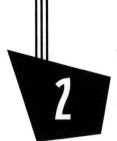

What Is It?
Asthma Defined

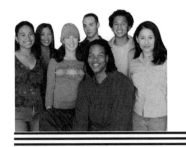

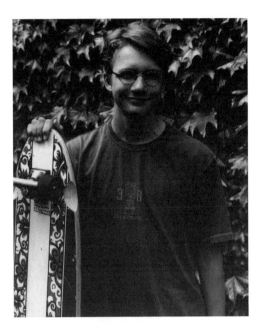

Torrey

Photo:
Penny Paquette

"When you are having an asthma attack, it feels like you are breathing through a small straw. When that happens, I sit down and try to pace my breathing. It feels like someone is closing the pipe to restrict the air coming into my lungs. . . . Occasionally, it affects my sports, but it has never kept me from playing."

Torrey is 14 years old. He likes to skate, play lacrosse, and ride bikes with his friends.

It feels like an elephant is sitting on my chest. I can't stop coughing. . . . It feels like my lungs are clogged and they are filled with glop. When my asthma is acting up, I just feel really tired. My chin itches. I just don't have the energy to walk to school. . . . I feel like my chest is full and I can't take a deep breath. When I laugh a lot, I start to wheeze.

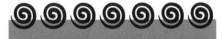

ASTHMA SYMPTOMS

- Chronic coughing
- Difficulty breathing
- Chest tightness
- Shortness of breath
- Wheezing

Asthma symptoms vary. If you think you may have asthma, see your doctor.

This is how young people describe what having asthma feels like. These feelings are common during asthma attacks. Wheezing, a tightening in the chest, difficulty breathing, and coughing are all symptoms of asthma. The information provided here will help you better understand asthma and its symptoms. It is not intended to help you treat yourself. Only a doctor can make a diagnosis of asthma, and because it is a serious disease, if you have these symptoms you should see your doctor or an asthma specialist.

Asthma symptoms provide a lot of information about what is happening in your body during an asthma attack. Because asthma is an illness that creates problems in the airways of the lungs, people with asthma often have trouble breathing. The symptoms are usually temporary, but some people require emergency services during an asthma episode.

According to the National Institutes of Health (NIH), asthma is a chronic inflammatory disorder of the airways. It is caused by swelling (inflammation). If you have asthma, your lungs are sensitive and your airways may swell when you are exposed to things that irritate them. When the airways are irritated, they react more aggressively than those of people without asthma. Doctors call this type of reaction hyperresponsiveness. That means your body overreacts, causing your airways to swell and fill with mucus.

NORMAL LUNG FUNCTION

When you breathe, air enters your respiratory system through your nose or mouth and travels down your trachea through your bronchial tubes. These bronchial airways help bring oxygen into your lungs and then to the tiny alveoli that carry the oxygen to the rest of your body. If you imagine this part of your respiratory system as a tree turned upside down, it is easy to picture what the system looks like. The trachea becomes the trunk of the tree, the bronchial tubes the main branches. These then branch out further to the smaller airways called bronchioles. At the end of the bronchioles are the alveoli, the tiny sacs that are responsible for making the air exchanges that carry oxygen into your body and carbon dioxide out. Inside the airways are tiny hairs that wiggle and wave and help wash inhaled particles out of the airways and into the throat. Once there, they are swallowed or coughed up. When this system is working breathing is easy.

ASTHMATIC BREATHING

If you have asthma, these airways can become what some doctors call hyperresponsive or twitchy. The tubes may swell or the muscles that make up the tubes may go into spasms and tighten. Doctors call this bronchoconstriction. This twitching and tightening makes the air-flow space much smaller or restricted. To make matters worse, sometimes cells in the tubes secrete a thick, sticky mucus that makes breathing even more difficult. The fluid is so thick that the tiny hairs within the airways can't clear it away. With the airways tightened and filled with mucus, they become more and more irritated making it more and more difficult to breathe. Often there is a whistling noise as the person struggles to pass air into or out of these hyperresponsive, inflamed, and irritated airways.

Imagine a drinking straw. You sip from your soft drink and the fluid is delivered into your mouth. Now imagine a pinched straw. The space is now narrowed and it is difficult to get the fluid into the straw. When an asthma attack occurs,

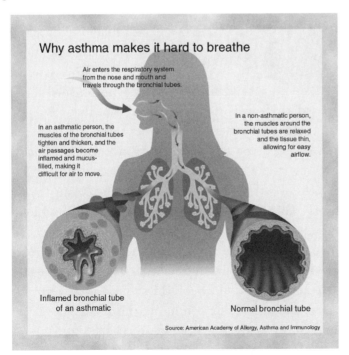

**Poster provided by the American Academy
of Asthma, Allergy, and Immunology**

the airways are pinched and it becomes difficult to get air into and out of the lungs. This restriction in the airways sometimes creates a wheezing noise often associated with asthma. Now imagine that in addition to being pinched, the straw is filled with thick honey. The honey represents the mucus that collects in an asthmatic's airways. Those with asthma cough in an attempt to clear the airways of the mucus.

Because airways are naturally narrower when we exhale, asthma makes exhaling extremely difficult. As the airways narrow during an asthma attack, it becomes impossible to completely exhale. The airways remain filled with the trapped air and new air can't enter. This is what causes that tight feeling in the chest and the shortness of breath that many asthmatics describe during an attack.

HOW IT FEELS

Imagine a long balloon with rubber bands tightened around it. That's what the muscles around the bronchiole do during an asthma attack.

If you have asthma, you know what that feels like. If you don't, try this experiment. Take a deep breath. Without exhaling, try to take in more air. Try again. Your breathing will become very shallow. That full and tight feeling mimics what it feels like to have an asthma attack. Fortunately, you can exhale and the symptoms will disappear. For asthmatics, it's not that easy.

Though many other lung diseases don't respond well to treatment, the good news is that asthma symptoms can be reversed. Asthma specialist Dr. Paul Hannaway says a good definition of asthma is "*reversible* obstructive airways disease." This long description can be remembered by the abbreviation ROAD. Sometimes the obstruction reverses on its own, but most often those with asthma must take medicine to prevent the asthma attack or to *reverse* it if it has already started. Although the symptoms can be reversed, the underlying condition, the airway inflammation, is always there.

Asthma symptoms usually come and go. If you have asthma and you have a good treatment plan, you may seldom have symptoms. Still, most asthmatics experience problems under certain circumstances. When asthmatics begin to cough and to wheeze and have trouble breathing, these episodes are most commonly called asthma attacks. Doctors sometimes call them exacerbations or flares. Although these attacks can come on suddenly, often there are warnings. As lung function diminishes, the body doesn't get enough oxygen. When you are deprived of oxygen, fatigue is often a warning sign. Asthma attacks can be mild, moderate, or severe. Sometimes one attack is followed by what doctors call a "second wave." Although asthma symptoms seemed to be back under control, a second and more serious attack can make breathing more difficult. Second waves are more serious and leave your airways even more sensitive. Sometimes, second wave attacks require a stay in the hospital.

Those with seasonal allergies may have problems at predictable times of the year. The onset of cold weather is a predictor of problems ahead for some asthmatics. Medical breathing devices can help predict coming asthma problems. Breathing can be monitored with a special device called a peak flow meter. This gadget can actually monitor breathing by measuring how well air flows out of the lungs. Lowered air-flow levels indicate spasms or inflammation in your bronchial airways, helping you recognize breathing problems even before you may feel them.

Although asthma exacerbations are often episodic and the symptoms can be reversed, the underlying condition, the airway inflammation, continues.

WHO GETS ASTHMA

Babies, children, teenagers, adults, and the elderly can all have asthma. Today, more than 17 million Americans have been diagnosed with the disease. Nearly one-third of those with asthma are under 18. It is the most common chronic childhood disease, affecting more than one child in twenty. The next time you are in a large group of young people, look around. If there are one hundred people in the group, at least five of them probably have asthma. So, if you have asthma, you are not alone.

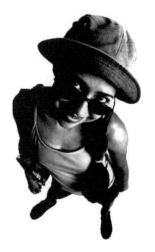

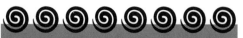

FAMOUS PEOPLE WITH ASTHMA

- Jason Alexander, actor
- Donovan Bailey, Canadian Olympic runner
- Ludwig von Beethoven, composer
- Leonard Bernstein, American composer, conductor, and pianist
- Jerome Bettis, football player and 2002 Walter Payton NFL Man of the Year
- Ambrose Bierce, author
- Calvin Coolidge, 30th President of the United States
- Coolio, Grammy-award-winning rap artist
- E. J. Corey, Nobel prize winner
- Dani, Sesame Street muppet
- Bruce Davidson, US Olympic equestrian
- Jim Davis, cartoonist, creator of Garfield
- Charles Dickens, author
- Tom Dolan, US Olympic medalist, swimming
- Sharon Donnelly, Canadian Olympic triathlete
- Vincent Damian Furnier (Alice Cooper), American rock musician and performer
- Kenneth Gorelick (Kenny G), musician and composer
- Kurte Grote, US Olympic medalist, swimming
- Ernesto (Che) Guevara, Argentine physician and freedom fighter
- Nancy Hogshead, US Olympic medalist, swimming
- Jim "Catfish" Hunter, baseball player
- Robert Joffrey, dancer and choreographer

Among the 17 million Americans with asthma are television stars, professional athletes, scientists, musicians, singers, directors, writers, and politicians. Although the famous bring attention to the disease, the not-so-famous have asthma, too. Firemen, plumbers, stockbrokers, teachers, at-home moms, lawyers, doctors, little league players, coaches, receptionists, telephone operators, and mechanics are also among those who have asthma.

More boys than girls have asthma as young children; among teenagers both boys and girls are affected in equal numbers.

Although asthma affects all races, it is slightly more prevalent among African Americans and Hispanics and among those who live in inner cities. Researchers believe that poverty is responsible for this finding. Rodents, insects, air pollution, as well as unaffordable heath care make asthma a greater problem for the poor. Most alarming is the fact that deaths from asthma are more likely for African Americans than for Caucasians.

HOW DO YOU GET IT?

Asthma is not contagious. You can't catch it from your friends. Heredity seems to play a factor as those with parents or siblings who have asthma are more likely to develop the disease. If one or both of your parents have allergies, your chances of developing asthma also increase. New research indicates several specific genes may be involved in asthma.

Smoking has been liked to asthma, and second-hand smoke may contribute to as many as 26,000 new cases of asthma each year. Although no one should smoke, it is especially dangerous if you have asthma. This includes marijuana as well. You can read more about this in chapter 4.

Viral infections in young children may also be responsible for asthma. Respiratory Syncytial Virus (RSV) can cause diseases in the bronchial system. If you had RSV as a child, you are especially vulnerable to developing asthma.

Asthma can be a debilitating disease. Among children, it is the leading cause of school absences—10 million a year. Ten million school days! Although a day off from school might sound like fun, those home with asthma often have to stay in bed and are too tired to enjoy themselves.

Although asthma is a treatable disease, it shouldn't be taken lightly. More than 5,000 people die from asthma each year. Asthma deaths are rare in children compared to the number of young people who have the disease. Still, young people do die each year. In 1993, 340 young people (under the age of 25) died from asthma. In most of these deaths, patients and their parents had little understanding of the disease or failed to recognize the danger signs associated with a serious asthma attack. If you have asthma, you need to work with your parents and your doctor to keep your asthma under control. Up until now, your parents have probably directly supervised your medications. As a young adult, you need to accept more of that responsibility. You are away from home more than when you were a young child and you are often involved in activities without adult supervision. You need to understand your asthma and take responsibility for monitoring your symptoms. If you would like to know

FAMOUS PEOPLE WITH ASTHMA
(Continued)

- Jackie Joyner-Kersee, US Olympic medalist, track and field
- John F. Kennedy, 35th President of the United States
- Bill Koch, US Olympic medalist, cross-country skiing
- Tseng Kuo-Fan, Chinese statesman, general, and scholar
- Liza Minnelli, singer and actress
- Walter Mondale, 42nd Vice-President of the United States
- Ernest (Dutch) Morial, American political, legal, and civil rights leader
- George Murray, Boston Marathon winner, wheelchair division
- Apolo Anton Ohno, US Olympic medalist, short track speed skating
- Peter the Great, Russian Czar
- Pliny the Elder, Roman historian and scholar
- Marcel Proust, novelist
- Joseph Pulitzer, publisher and philanthropist
- Gary Roberts, Toronto Maple Leafs hockey player
- Dennis Rodman, basketball player
- Theodore Roosevelt, 26th President of the United States
- Martin Scorsese, film director
- William Tecumseh Sherman, Civil War general
- Elizabeth Taylor, actress
- Amy Van Dyken, US Olympic medalist, swimming
- Bonnie Warner, American luge specialist
- Dominique Wilkins, basketball player

more about monitoring and controlling your asthma symptoms, read chapter 5.

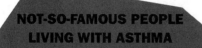

NOT-SO-FAMOUS PEOPLE LIVING WITH ASTHMA

➤ Me
➤ My daughter
➤ My son
➤ My grandson
➤ You?

Asthma attacks can be triggered by a variety of causes including specific allergies such as pollens and pets; irritants such as smoke or specific odors like paint, cleaning products, cooking smells, or perfumes; infections including colds, sinus infections, and the flu; changes in temperature; heartburn; and exercise. This is just a brief list of some asthma triggers. There is more information on this subject in chapter 4.

For some young people, symptoms decrease with age. Some teenagers who had asthma as children are no longer troubled by asthma symptoms. Others find their symptoms return during their teen years. If you are a teenager and have asthma now, it is likely that you will continue to have it as an adult.

ASTHMA ON THE RISE

The incidence of asthma is increasing. Although researchers aren't sure what is responsible for the increase, there are several theories. Dr. Calman Prussin, head of the clinical allergy and immunology unit at the National Institute of Allergy and Infectious Diseases (NIAID), believes asthma may be on the rise because people are spending more time indoors. In a recent release from NIAID, Dr. Prussin said, "Our houses are now hermetically sealed to save heating and cooling energy, and unfortunately this causes more indoor allergen exposure." Increased levels of air pollution, inadequate exercise, and rising obesity may also play a role in the asthma increase according to Dr. Prussin.

The American Medical Association (AMA) believes several other factors are playing a role in the rising numbers. The increased survival of premature infants with underdeveloped lungs may play a role in the increasing rates. Women who smoke when they are pregnant or around their young children may also be contributing to the increased incidence. Poverty also plays a role. Those living

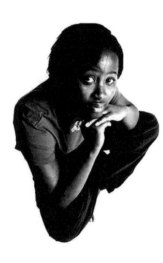

in poverty are frequently exposed to urban air pollution, rodents, and insects that make asthma worse.

Some researchers believe that our quest to be clean, to reduce our exposure to germs, and to become immune to disease may be backfiring. Our cleanliness quest may be responsible for the increases in asthma and allergies. Researchers have been exploring the possibility since the late 1980s when a British epidemiologist reported that smaller families had fewer infections, but a higher incidence of asthma and allergies. The reduced exposure to germs provides infants with fewer opportunities to fight off infections and their inexperienced immune systems become lazy and more likely to develop allergic responses to seemingly harmless substances like pollen or dust.

Evidence of this "hygiene hypothesis" mounted when studies of infants in day care centers produced unexpected findings. While day care babies under 6 months had higher rates of illness including asthma, those same children were 40 percent less likely to have asthma by the time they were between 6 and 12 years old. This makes researchers suspect that those exposed to germs at an early age get an immune system boost that helps prevent allergies and asthma as they get older.

> Some researchers believe we are too clean. They call this theory the hygiene hypothesis.

In addition to the exposure to germs, exposure to a special form of dust may also help. House dust that contains endotoxins, a chemical present in part of the cell wall of live and dead bacteria, may help protect against asthma and allergies. According to Dr. Andy Liu, a pediatric allergy and asthma specialist at the National Jewish Medical and Research Center, house dust endotoxin is significantly higher in rural areas or developing countries where asthma and allergies are less prevalent. Researchers at the research center used this information when studying the effects of endotoxin exposure in Denver. They discovered that endotoxin levels were much lower in the homes of children with allergies and asthma than their non-wheezy control group. Early exposure to this type of dust seems to steer the immune system down a non-allergic pathway according to Dr. Liu.

Although this type of exposure early in life may help prevent allergies and asthma, researchers caution that those already allergic or sensitive to dust should keep their homes as dust free as possible.

FAST FACTS

- ▶ More than 17 million Americans have asthma.
- ▶ 4.8 million teenagers and children have asthma.
- ▶ Young people are hospitalized 200,000 times each year because of asthma.
- ▶ Asthmatic teens and children miss 10 million days of school.
- ▶ Asthma is slightly more prevalent among blacks and inner-city residents.
- ▶ Worldwide, asthma has doubled within the past 15 years.
- ▶ There is no cure for asthma.
- ▶ With treatment, asthmatics can lead a normal life.

QUICK REVIEW

Asthma is a disease that causes swelling in the airways and makes breathing difficult. It affects millions of people. Although breathing is sometimes difficult for asthmatics, the symptoms can be treated. To learn more about the different types of asthma, how it is diagnosed, asthma triggers and treatments, and what you can do about your asthma, read on.

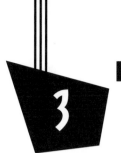

Diagnosing Asthma

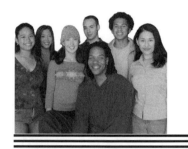

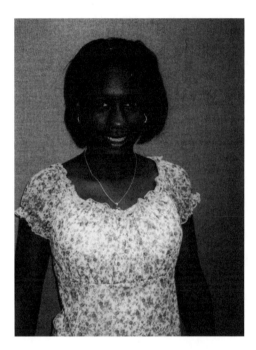

Chemise

Photo: Penny Paquette

"I have problems when running, in soccer, when cheering, and jumping around. My chest hurts and I feel short of breath."

Despite her exercise-induced asthma, Chemise, a sophomore in high school, is a cheerleader, a runner, and a soccer player. She says, "Be careful. Take care of yourself. Dress warm in the winter. Do lots of sports."

If you have the symptoms discussed in the previous chapter, you may have asthma. Remember though, you don't need to have all the symptoms to have asthma. Not everyone with asthma wheezes. Not everyone with asthma coughs. Maybe you have symptoms only when you are exercising or doing heavy work. Maybe you only cough at night. Some teenagers have asthma symptoms all of the time, but for most, asthma is episodic. It comes and goes. If you have asthma symptoms, talk to your doctor.

Many teens with asthma don't realize they have it. They think they are out of shape, have a cold, or a lingering infection. It is unfortunate that so many with asthma go undiagnosed. Some studies have shown that up to half of those with asthma are undiagnosed. Without a diagnosis, they don't get treatment, and without treatment, they can't get better.

If you suspect you have asthma, you need to make an appointment to see your doctor. Your family pediatrician or family doctor can diagnose asthma, or your doctor may send you to a specialist if he or she suspects you may have asthma. Allergy and asthma specialists treat allergic disorders as well as asthma, and pulmonologists diagnose and treat asthma as well as other diseases of the lungs. You can seek help from your family physician, but if you still have symptoms and/or your treatment is not helping, you may want to seek out a specialist. According to the American Medical Association's (AMA) asthma guide, recent studies showed that both general physicians and asthma specialists were equally effective in treating those with mild asthma. For those with more severe asthma, however, specialists provided better treatment results. Those with asthma who worked with specialists missed fewer days from work and school, they had fewer hospital visits, and they had fewer relapses.

The AMA recommends seeing a specialist if:

◎ **you have ever had a life threatening episode**

◎ **your asthma symptoms do not decrease within three to six months of treatment**

◎ **you have nasal polyps, gastric reflux (heartburn), or chronic sinus infections that make your asthma worse**

◎ **you need special testing such as skin testing, bronchoscopy, or an allergy challenge (see below)**

◎ **there is confusion over your diagnosis**

◎ **your symptoms appear to be allergy related**

◎ **you need help to stop smoking or you need to control irritants in your environment**

◎ **a child younger than three has severe asthma**

◎ **your asthma is triggered by your job or an environmental hazard that requires special attention**

HISTORY OF ALLERGY TESTING

Until the late 1800s, there were no specific tests for allergies. The Ancient Egyptians knew allergies existed and were the first to record an allergic reaction when a pharaoh died of a wasp sting. In the 1500s, Girolamo Cardano suspected the Archbishop of Scotland was allergic to the feathers in his pillow and mattress. The doctor suggested that the Archbishop remove the feathers. Consequently, his asthma improved.

But, it wasn't until 1873 that allergies could be confirmed by skin testing. Dr. Charles Blackley performed the first skin test for allergies when he scraped his arm and then rubbed pollen into the scratch. He recorded his reaction as a hive or wheal at the scratch site.

Later in the early 1900s Drs. Noon and Freeman began diagnosing those with allergies by putting drops of allergens into their patients' eyes. The patients' eyes would tear, swell, or get red if they were allergic to the substance. They then treated the allergic patients with the first allergy shots designed to help patients develop a tolerance to allergens.

Depending on the severity of your asthma and the type of insurance plan your family has, a specialist may design a treatment plan and have your general physician help you follow the plan, or the specialist may take over.

Your doctor can recommend a specialist, or your health insurance may have specialists that are part of your health care plan. Your local hospital may have a list of specialists who treat asthma. The American Academy of Allergy Asthma and Immunology website provides a list of specialists in your area (www.aaaai.org) and the American Lung Association in your area can provide lists of specialists. Your parents can make the necessary appointments and get your asthma symptoms evaluated.

FAMILY HISTORY

The doctor will probably begin by collecting information about your general health and your family's health history. As your doctor explores your family history, your symptoms, and runs tests, he or she will not only be diagnosing asthma, but eliminating other conditions with similar symptoms (see following sidebar).

Common symptoms of asthma include wheezing, chest tightness, shortness of breath, coughing, excessive mucus, and fatigue. Sinus infections, sinus headaches, and bronchitis are often associated with asthma as well. You may want to keep a record of your symptoms and the conditions contributing to your symptoms before you go to the doctor. For example, if you wheeze when running, write that down. If you cough during the night, but feel better in the morning, write that down. If you seem to be most affected in the cold, write that down. If you are bothered only in the fall, spring, or winter, make a note of that. If you have a new job or you are exposed to chemicals or latex at work, record that in your notes. Your doctor will want to know if any foods or beverages make your symptoms worse, if your symptoms get worse in a particular location, and whether you have pets at home. If you make notes about the conditions that affect your asthma, it will give the doctor the information needed to evaluate your symptoms.

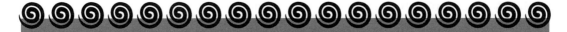

ILLNESSES THAT MAY SEEM LIKE ASTHMA

Several airway diseases have symptoms that mimic asthma. Like asthma, these diseases cause problems with breathing and many cause the wheezing noise associated with asthma.

BRONCHIECTASIS (PRONOUNCED BRON-KEE-ECK-TAH-IS)

Bronchiectasis is a rare condition that affects the lungs. The bronchial tubes become enlarged and distorted, forming pockets. Mucus collects and clogs these pockets and causes more damage to the airways. The tiny hairs that line the bronchial tubes and help clear them of dust, germs, and mucus are destroyed. These clogged pockets are very susceptible to infections. Large amounts of foul smelling pus collects and a chronic cough develops in an attempt to clear away the phlegm.

Bronchiectasis can be caused by infections in the bronchial walls, immune deficiencies, or cystic fibrosis (see below). Sometimes severe heartburn can cause stomach acids to be inhaled, irritating the bronchial tubes. Obstructions can also cause the condition. Sometimes young children inhale a small food particle that clears the windpipe, but blocks a small airway. The blockage damages the airway and allows an infection to develop.

The major symptom is a chronic cough, and people with bronchiectasis can cough up large amounts of phlegm. Sometimes they may cough up blood as well.

Antibiotics can help clear the infection and bronchodilator medicines can help relax the airways. Medicines that control heartburn may be recommended. If a foreign object is causing the problem, it needs to be removed.

Patients need to use what doctors call "postural drainage" to help clear the lungs and bronchial tubes. The patient hangs his or her head over the side of the bed, leaving the lung area above the head. This allows gravity to do some of the work the bronchial tubes can no longer do and helps clear the airways. Clapping on the chest with hands or exhaling into a specialized device can also help clear the mucus. If treatment is ineffective, surgery is occasionally suggested.

BRONCHITIS

As in asthma, airways are blocked and clogged with mucus in bronchitis. The trachea and bronchial tubes are inflamed and may create the wheezing sound often associated with asthma. Bronchitis can be caused by a viral infection or by bacteria. It can also come from inhaling irritants like cigarette smoke, dust, or chemicals.

Acute or short-term bronchitis may follow a head cold that develops into a chest cold. It usually goes away in a few days. People with asthma can also have bronchitis, and it can make asthma symptoms worse.

Chronic bronchitis, a chronic obstructive pulmonary disease (COPD), develops slowly over time. Airways can become irritated and thick following long-term exposure to irritants. Mucus is produced constantly and a chronic cough develps. Chemicals and fumes can contribute to chronic bronchitis, but the most common cause is cigarette smoke.

(Continued)

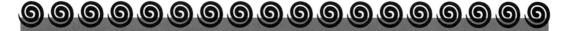

ILLNESSES THAT MAY SEEM LIKE ASTHMA *(Continued)*

Once the airways are irritated, swollen, and filled with mucus, infections often set in. The infection can be treated with antibiotics, but the inflammation, thickening, mucus, and cough don't go away. There are medicines than can improve the situation, but the underlying condition continues. The best treatment for chronic bronchitis is to avoid the irritant. Anyone who smokes is at risk of developing chronic bronchitis.

CYSTIC FIBROSIS (CF)

Cystic Fibrosis is an inherited genetic disease of the mucus glands that affects children and young adults. With cystic fibrosis, the body produces excessive amounts of thick, sticky mucus that block the airway, damage the lungs, and lead to infection. CF also affects the ability to digest food.

The symptoms of CF can be similar to asthma as they can include wheezing, coughing, and excessive mucus, but CF can also cause poor weight gain, persistent diarrhea, and salty-tasting skin.

Doctors can diagnose CF with a test called the sweat test. It measures the amount of salt in the sweat. Those with CF usually have high salt levels.

As with bronchitis, mucus drainage can be improved with postural drainage and chest percussions, and antiobiotics can be used to treat infections. When CF affects the digestive system, patients need to eat enriched diets and take vitamins and enzymes.

Mucus thinners, bronchodilator medicines, and decongestants are used to improve breathing.

CF is frequently fatal. On average, those with CF live to be about 30 years old. Doctors identified the CF gene in 1989 and continue to explore gene therapy as a way to prevent or cure CF, as well as drug therapies that may help treat CF.

EMPHYSEMA

Emphysema, like chronic bronchitis, is a COPD. It destroys the smallest airways that empty into air sacs called alveoli. The alveoli become overinflated and eventually break down or collapse. That reduces the number of normal air sacs. The damaged and reduced air sacs are no longer able to get adequate oxygen into the bloodstream. This causes the lungs to lose their elasticity, leading to what is sometimes called floppy airways.

Those with emphysema have trouble moving air into and out of their lungs. The respiratory muscles struggle to bring adequate oxygen to the body and to remove carbon dioxide. Emphysema can lead to heart failure.

Shortness of breath is a common symptom of emphysema. Unfortunately, those with emphysema have lost 50 to 70 percent of their lung tissue by the time they develop symptoms. As the disease worsens, symptoms can include fatigue and weight loss. The continued struggle to breathe results in a barrel-chested appearance and overdeveloped neck and shoulder muscles.

(Continued)

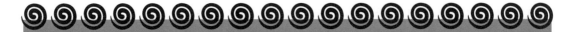

ILLNESSES THAT MAY SEEM LIKE ASTHMA *(Continued)*

Lung function tests like those used to diagnose asthma are also used to diagnose emphysema.

Up to 90 percent of emphysema is caused by smoking. Some with emphysema, however, have a protein deficiency that may lead to an inherited form of emphysema.

Emphysema cannot be cured, but those who quit smoking can slow its progress. Bronchodilator drugs that relax air passages can help reduce symptoms; antibiotics can treat infections; and specialized drugs are available for those with the inherited form of emphysema.

Lung volume reduction surgery and lung transplant are high-risk procedures that can be effective.

CONGESTIVE HEART FAILURE

Congestive Heart Failure happens when the heart loses its pumping ability and can no longer adequately deliver enough blood to the lungs and the rest of the body. The weakened pumping action causes fluid to collect in the lungs.

The first symptom of congestive heart failure is usually shortness of breath with exercise. Gradually, however, even minor exertion can create breathing problems. Eventually those with congestive heart failure have trouble breathing even at rest. Swollen ankles and feet, fatigue, a persistent cough, and wheezing are also symptoms of congestive heart failure.

Because some of the symptoms are similar to those of asthma, this condition is sometimes called cardiac asthma.

Treatment includes medicines to reduce fluid retention and increase lung action. Angiotensin converting enzyme (ACE) inhibitors are also used to treat heart disease. Lifestyle changes can prolong life as well. Weight control, not smoking, eating well, and avoiding alcoholic drinks can help.

The outlook for those with congestive heart failure depends on age, the severity of the problem, general heath, and other factors. About two-thirds of those diagnosed with congestive heart failure die within five years. Some, however, live longer, even into old age.

VOCAL CORD DYSFUNCTION (VCD)

Vocal Cord Dysfunction is sometimes called laryngeal asthma. According to the National Jewish Medical and Research Center, which specializes in respiratory diseases, nearly 25 percent of the patients referred to them with a diagnosis of asthma actually have VCD.

With VCD, the vocal cords may decrease in size by 10 to 40 percent. This restriction may create trouble breathing, difficulty swallowing, and a choking sensation. The abnormal action of the vocal chords can cause a wheezing noise often associated with asthma.

Diagnosis must be made by viewing the vocal cords. Treatment includes speech therapy, relaxation techniques, and psychotherapy. Severe attacks may be treated with a mixture of helium and oxygen.

Because asthma and allergies often run in families, your doctor will ask not only about your symptoms, but illnesses in other family members. If you or members of your family have asthma or allergies, that presents another risk factor for the condition. If one of your parents has asthma, you have a 50 percent chance of having it, too. If both of your parents have asthma, you have a whopping 75 percent chance of having asthma as well. Maybe none of your siblings or your parents have allergies or asthma, but your grandparents do. Your doctor will want to know that. If you or family members have rhinitis or hay fever, or if anyone has eczema, your doctor will want to know that, too.

Your doctor will give you a routine physical exam and check your heart and lungs. If you are having problems breathing or the doctor can hear wheezing or coughing, that information will contribute to the diagnostic puzzle. The doctor will listen as you inhale and as you exhale. When airways are obstructed, your doctor may hear a wheezing sound. Those with asthma have swelling in their breathing tubes that narrows the airways like a squeezed straw. When you breath out, it may take longer for you to expel air than for those who have clear breathing tubes. Your doctor will have you take shallow breaths and deep breaths. Sometimes asthma symptoms can be triggered by deep breathing even if normal breathing doesn't cause problems.

Your doctor will look at your rib cage. Those with asthma often have differences in the shape of their ribs resulting from the way they breathe. This is often described as a barrel-chested appearance.

The doctor will examine your skin for signs of hives, eczema, or other skin irritations that may be allergy related. He or she will check your ears, your eyes, and your nose as well. Ear blockages, sinus problems, and itchy eyes can all be clues in diagnosing asthma.

PULMONARY FUNCTION TESTS

One of the most common tests used to diagnose asthma is a pulmonary function test. This test presents information that helps in the diagnosis, and helps measure the severity of asthma. Because the expected results of the test are based on size and age, the doctor will weigh and measure you or ask for your age, height, and weight.

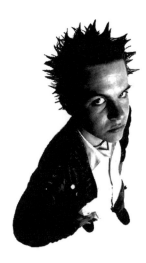

Your doctor will have you blow into a device called a spirometer, which will measure the amount of air and the speed at which you can exhale. This test doesn't hurt. The doctor or nurse will place a disposable cardboard tube into the tubing on the machine and have you blow into it as forcefully as you can to empty your lungs. You will blow hard into the machine until your lungs are completely empty. This helps your doctor measure the maximum amount of air your lungs can hold (vital capacity or VC), the maximum rate of airflow that you can generate when you force the air out (peak expiratory flow rate or PEFR), and how much air you can blow out in one second (forced expiratory volume or FEV). The doctor will compare your performance results with those of healthy individuals your age and size.

This forceful breathing often causes increased symptoms in those who have asthma. You may cough or wheeze after the test. The doctor or nurse may have you breathe a medicine designed to open your bronchial tubes and then repeat the test. Often those with asthma perform better after being pretreated with this medicine before breathing into the spirometer. The breathing improvement indicates that the asthma symptoms are reversible and is a sign that you probably have asthma.

Not everyone with asthma improves after using the medicine, however. Some have air tubes that are so tight that the medicine cannot penetrate their bronchial tubes to relax them. If you fall into this category, you may need to be treated with an asthma medicine for several weeks before being retested for signs of improvement. Again, improvement after treatment is an indication that you have asthma.

Some have mild asthma symptoms or episodic symptoms that may not affect breathing results during spirometer test. If this is the case, the doctor may give you a test designed to provoke symptoms. For many people with asthma, exercise can provoke symptoms. Your doctor may have you exercise by running on a treadmill or riding a stationary bike. He or she will measure your breathing before you start with a small handheld device called a peak flow meter that measures how fast you can empty your lungs, or your PEFR. (More about this device in chapter 5.) The doctor or nurse will take another reading while you exercise and perhaps another when you finish exercising. Most young people with asthma show reductions in their airflow within ten minutes of exercising.

Another test that is sometimes used in those who have normal breathing results on the spirometer is called a challenge test. The doctor will have you breathe a mist of a chemical known to provoke asthma called methacholine. It can take a very little bit of this chemical to provoke asthma symptoms in those with severe problems—more in those with less severe asthma. If your lung function falls by 20 percent following the challenge test, asthma is most likely the cause. If your lung function falls following the test, the doctor or nurse will give you an inhaled medicine to reverse the symptoms and relax your airway muscles. Those with no reaction to the chemical probably do not have asthma.

If an allergy is suspected as a trigger, your doctor may order blood tests and skin tests to help identify specific allergens. A blood test can detect the presence of immunoglobulin E (IgE) antibodies that may indicate an allergy. Your blood test may also show allergy cells or eosinophils. A small blood sample is taken and sent off to the lab for examination.

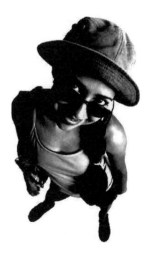

Your doctor may also order skin tests to help identify specific allergies that may be causing asthma symptoms. There are many allergies that can trigger asthma. Skin tests can determine if you are allergic to specific allergens such as dust, trees, pets, etc. Although a positive allergy test does not necessarily mean you have asthma, it does indicate a risk factor for asthma and helps identify triggers that may be causing your symptoms. Dust mites, animal proteins, mold, pollen, and cockroaches can all produce allergic reactions in sensitive people. Some people are allergic to insect stings, foods, latex, and certain drugs. You can read more about allergies as asthma triggers in chapter 4.

Prick or scratch tests, called percutaneous tests, are the most common methods for exploring allergy sensitivity. A tiny amount of specific allergen is scratched or pricked into the skin. In people with allergies, special IgE antibodies activate special cells called mast cells. These cells then release chemicals that doctors call mediators. The chemical causes redness, swelling, and/or itching. If you are allergic to specific allergens, only the areas that were scratched with that allergen will react and you will get a small hive or swollen spot where that allergen was scratched into your skin. If you are not allergic to the specific allergen pricked into the skin, that area will not react. Reaction time usually happens within 15 minutes, so doctors can quickly find out what you are allergic to and then help develop a plan to avoid that allergen.

If your prick tests are not clear, your doctor may give you an intradermal test. Instead of simply scratching the skin with specific allergens, the doctor will inject them just under skin. Again, if you are allergic to a specific allergen, your skin will swell, get red, and/or itch at the injection site.

Sometimes people taking certain medications, those with skin conditions, or very young children are not good candidates for prick or intradermal tests. In that case, doctors often use a special blood test called a RAST test or radioallergosorbent test. The nurse or technician will clean your skin and then insert a needle in your arm that is attached to a collecting tube. Your blood will be sent to the lab to be analyzed. At the lab, technicians will test samples of your blood with specific allergens. If you are allergic to a particular substance, IgE antibodies will attach to the substance indicating you are allergic to it. Doctors can use the results of this test to determine exactly what you are allergic to and then develop an avoidance or treatment strategy to help you.

OTHER TESTS

If your breathing tests are inconclusive, or if you have other symptoms your doctor would like to examine further, your doctor may then order additional tests to help diagnose asthma and to rule out other problems that may have similar symptoms. X-rays can help eliminate disorders with similar symptoms such as emphysema, pneumonia, and bronchitis. Depending on your age and general health, your doctor may also need to rule out respiratory tract infections, blood clots in your lungs, heart failure, and tumors.

If you are having problems with your sinuses, your doctor may also order diagnostic x-rays or CAT scans of your sinus areas.

SEVERITY CLASSIFICATIONS

Doctors use a standardized system of classifying the severity of asthma. Your symptoms and the regularity of those symptoms help your doctor define the type of asthma you have. The type of symptoms you experience, how often your experience them, how much they get in the way of your daily activities, and how much they disrupt your nights help determine how your doctor will classify your asthma. The frequency and the severity of your asthma attacks or what the National Heart, Lung, and Blood

ASTHMA CLASSIFICATION ACCORDING TO SEVERITY

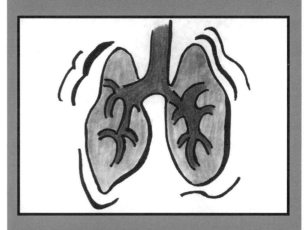

Mild Intermittent

- ▶ **Symptoms are infrequent and occur less often than two times a week**
- ▶ **Symptoms or "flare-ups" last a few hours to a few days**
- ▶ **Nighttime symptoms are infrequent; fewer than twice a month**
- ▶ **Peak flow readings are higher than 80 percent**
- ▶ **Rapid-acting bronchodilator inhaler taken as needed**

Mild Persistent

- ▶ **Symptoms occur more than twice a week, but not daily**
- ▶ **Episodes may affect activities**
- ▶ **Nighttime symptoms occur more than twice a month**
- ▶ **Peak flow readings greater than 80 percent**
- ▶ **Rapid-acting bronchodilator inhaler to control symptoms and low-dose inhaled corticosteroid (alternative treatment: cromolyn or leukotriene receptor antagonist)**

(Continued)

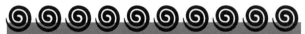

ASTHMA CLASSIFICATION ACCORDING TO SEVERITY (Continued)

Moderate Persistent

▶ Daily symptoms
▶ Flare-ups occur more than two times a week, lasting for several days
▶ Flare-ups may affect activities
▶ Nighttime symptoms occur more than once a week
▶ Peak flow readings between 60 and 80 percent
▶ Daily medication. Low-dose anti-inflammatory inhaler and long-acting inhaled beta-2 agonists or medium-dose inhaled anti-inflammatory and long-acting beta-2 agonists (alternative treatment: medium-dose inhaled corticosteroids and either leukotriene receptor antagonist or theophylline)

Severe Persistent

▶ Continual symptoms
▶ Flare-ups occur more than twice a week and may last for days
▶ Symptoms may interfere with daily activities; physical activities limited
▶ Nighttime symptoms are frequent
▶ Peak flow readings below 60 percent
▶ Multiple drug treatments may include high dose anti-inflammatory inhaler, long-acting beta-2 agonists, and if needed, oral corticosteriods

Note: Patients' treatments vary. Individual treatment plans should be developed with your doctor.

Classifications based on NHLBI, NIH recommendations.

Institute (NHLBI) call "exacerbations," also help doctors classify and treat your asthma. One of the measures doctors use in determining the severity of your asthma symptoms is your PEFR. You can read more about this in chapter 5. Once your doctor has reviewed your symptoms and the results of breathing tests, he or she will use the following guidelines to diagnose the severity of your asthma. The classifications are divided into four categories and your asthma classification may change classifications over time and/or following treatment.

Mild Intermittent

If your asthma symptoms occur only occasionally and last only a few hours or a day or two, you probably have what doctors call mild intermittent asthma. Readings on your peak flow meter fall into the 80 percent range during asthma episodes, but readings return to normal between episodes.

Mild Persistent

Those with mild persistent asthma have more "persistent" problems. If you have mild persistent asthma, you may experience shortness of breath, wheezing, and/or coughing more often than twice a week, but you don't experience symptoms every day. Your sleep may be disrupted by asthma symptoms a few times each month. Although your activities may be disrupted during episodes, you are able to return to normal activities once your symptoms have gone away. Readings on your peak flow meter will be in the 80 percent range and can vary by 20 to 30 percent. Your episodes may be provoked by specific triggers like cold air or exercise and may be treated with a fast-acting inhaler. Your doctor might recommend using an inhaler before exercise.

Moderate Persistent

As the name indicates, asthma symptoms occur more frequently and are more severe with moderate persistent asthma. If you fall into this category, you probably have some symptoms of asthma each day. You may wheeze, feel a tightness in your chest, cough, or feel short of breath at some point each day. The symptoms may get worse more than twice a week and your symptoms may last for several days. You may not be able to participate in your normal activities during these episodes. Readings on your peak flow meter will range from 60 to 80 percent and can vary as much as 30 percent.

Severe Persistent

As you might think, this is the most severe category. If you have asthma symptoms each day and flare-ups that last for extended periods, you may have severe persistent asthma. During these episodes, your daily activities and your physical activities are limited. You probably have trouble sleeping or wake up with symptoms. Your peak flow readings will fall below 60 percent and may vary as much as 30 percent.

Patients at any level of severity can have severe attacks, and if you have asthma, you need to consult a physician. Treatment plans are individualized not only according to severity, but according to the type or types of asthma you may have. There is more about treatment plans in chapter 5.

TYPES OF ASTHMA

Sometimes asthma is classified according to the causes, commonly called triggers, of asthma symptoms or an asthma attack. Not everyone who has asthma is affected by allergies. All asthmatics do not have hay fever. Some are most affected by physical exercise. As Moses Maimonides recognized in the 12th century, each asthmatic is different.

These categories may help you better understand your particular symptoms. Some people's symptoms fall into only one category, but for many, multiple categories apply. If you would like to know more about specific triggers, read chapter 4.

Extrinsic or Intrinsic?

Doctors sometimes use the term *extrinsic* asthma to describe asthma triggered by allergies. If you have asthma and allergies, your immune system produces a specific antibody, IgE, in response to exposure to an allergen. IgE sets off a series of responses causing the airways to become inflamed, to swell, and to produce mucus.

Those with *intrinsic* asthma have no history of allergies. Although doctors still don't know what causes this type of asthma, it often follows a respiratory virus infection.

It is important to know that no matter what type of asthma you have, the symptoms are created by the same factors, hyperresponsiveness, constriction, increased mucus, and inflammation.

Allergic Asthma

Teens with this type of extrinsic asthma have specific allergies that provoke asthma symptoms. Their symptoms are triggered by allergens. Pet dander, dust, and pollen are

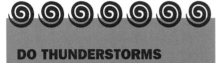

DO THUNDERSTORMS CAUSE ASTHMA?

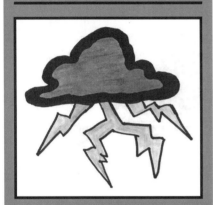

British researchers wondered the same thing. They set up a system of monitoring after-office-hour phone calls to doctors' answering services. They evaluated phone calls in a particular area on two different nights—one during clear weather and one during thunderstorm activity. On the night of the thunderstorm, doctors received 488 asthma-related phone calls. On the clear night, they only received 48!

Why the difference? They believe the high winds associated with storms can bring pollens into an area from far away creating large amounts of airborne allergens, provoking asthma symptoms in sensitive individuals.

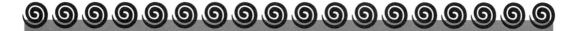

ITCHY SKIN—IT'S NOT A ZIT; IT'S AD

Although not everyone with eczema has asthma, many people with asthma also have eczema. In fact, eczema is associated with many allergic disorders including hay fever and food allergies. Most people who have eczema have had it since they were babies. Some outgrow it by the time they are two, but others continue to have problems through their teen years. Some people always have it.

Eczema is a general term for skin inflammations. Atopic dermatitis (AD) is the more precise medical term for the most severe and chronic skin disorder that causes extremely itchy, dry, inflamed skin. The skin can't hold enough moisture and becomes red, irritated, and sometimes weepy. Some people have patches of dry, thick, itchy skin that cracks and peels away. Doctors call these itchy patches lesions. These lesions tend to appear on the face, behind the ears, inside the elbow joint area, behind the knees, and on the buttocks. Weepy, crusted areas develop from scratching the lesions. Sometimes, these lesions become infected and are surrounded by pus-filled areas called pustules.

The skin condition runs in families. If one of your parents has AD, asthma, or hay fever, you have a one in four chance of developing it, too. If both parents have it, your chances are even higher. Still, about 30 percent of people with eczema have no family history of the skin condition.

Like asthma, AD symptoms can come and go. Some specific irritants can cause AD flares in some people, including many of the same triggers that provoke asthma symptoms. Solvents and cleaners, paints, astrigents and other alcohol-containing skin care products, soaps and detergents, perfumes, some cosmetics, fumes (including cigarette smoke), acidic foods, and woolens can irritate the skin of those with AD. Specific allergens, including foods like eggs, milk, nuts, wheat, some seafoods, or soy products, can make symptoms worse in sensitive individuals. Dust mites and pets may also be a factor.

People with AD have dry, brittle skin. It just won't stay moist enough to keep it from splitting and cracking. Winter months are particularly bad for most people with AD. Indoor heat and low humidity make the skin condition worse, but high humidity can cause problems, too. Sweating can make symptoms worse. Irritants, like those mentioned above, are also a factor for many. Emotional stress seems to make matters worse, too.

Treatment for AD begins with the underlying cause of the problem—dry skin. Keeping the skin moist can help prevent AD flares. Although there are many preparations out there to help with skin problems in teens, most contain alcohol and perfumes that can make matters worse if you have AD. The National Eczema Association recommends a very basic, inexpensive product for the treatment of dry skin conditions—petroleum jelly. Vaseline is probably the most recognized petroleum jelly product, but drugstores and grocery stores sell a variety of petroleum jelly products. They also recommend washing in warm, not hot water. Many teens believe scrubbing will help get rid of the patches on their skin. If you have AD, this can make problems worse. It is better to gently rub your skin and then blot with a towel to dry. It is best to apply moisturizer while your skin is still damp. Try not to scratch. Because AD can itch intensely, this is often very difficult. Try to keep your hands busy.

There are many topical prescription treatments available for AD flare-ups and for the skin infections often associated with them. Talk to your family doctor, an allergist, or a dermatologist about a treatment plan. They can also prescribe medicines to help with the itching.

just a few of the allergens that can affect people. If you have this type of asthma you may have a family history of allergies or a skin problem called eczema.

Seasonal Asthma

As the name indicates, some people have asthma in specific seasons. Allergies are also responsible for this type of asthma. If you have symptoms only in the spring when trees, grasses, and other plants are flowering, you may have this type of asthma. If a walk in the autumn leaves seem to provoke symptoms, you may also fall in this category.

Cold air seems to be a major asthma trigger for many people, so winters may be difficult. Exercising in cold weather can create a double-whammy especially for those who have exercise-induced asthma.

Exercise-Induced Asthma (EIA)

Many teenagers with asthma experience asthma symptoms with exercise. Some have allergies; some don't. Sometimes teenagers who don't normally exhibit asthma symptoms may experience asthma episodes during or following exercise.

Even the ancients recognized that asthma symptoms can come as a result of exercise. Arataeus the Cappadocian (200 A.D.) called the difficult breathing that sometimes follows exercise, asthma.

If you have never been diagnosed with asthma, but cough, wheeze, feel tight in the chest, or short of breath during or shortly following exercise, you may have exercise-induced asthma, or EIA. Those with EIA usually experience symptoms within five to twenty minutes of beginning to exercise or shortly after they stop exercising. In some cases, asthma symptoms may appear up to several hours after exercising. This type of asthma is often under diagnosed.

TIPS FOR EXERCISE-INDUCED ASTHMA
- Develop a plan with your doctor
- If recommended, use a pre-exercise medication
- Always take the time to warm up and cool down
- Cover your mouth and nose with a scarf when exercising in cold weather
- Choose the right sport for your symptoms

Sometimes coaches or gym teachers see this shortness of breath as a sign of being out of shape, and sometimes that is the case. But, many young people who experience difficulty breathing while exercising are not out of shape.

Even serious athletes can experience these symptoms. Studies by Dr. John Weiler of the American Academy of Allergy, Asthma and Immunology (AAAAI) and Edward Ryan of the United States Olympic Committee found that 44 of the 196 American athletes in the 1998 Winter Games had asthma. In the 1996 Summer Games in Atlanta, 1 in 6 American athletes had asthma. Studies prove that fitness is not a factor in EIA, and just as important, they show that asthma need not limit athletic pursuits.

Many Olympic competitors have asthma. In the 1998 Winter Games, 44 of 196 American athletes had asthma.

Cold air can be a factor, however. Although exercise-induced asthma can happen in any climate, EIA incidents are far more frequent when breathing cold, dry air.

In order to compete, athletes with EIA must be diagnosed and treated. "Yes, athletes who have asthma can compete at high levels," says Dr. Christopher Randolph, Chair of the AAAAI Sports Medicine Committee. "However, in order for these athletes to remain healthy and competitive, they must be diagnosed with asthma and take proper steps to control their condition."

Dr. Randolph believes that those with EIA have sensitive airways and their airways respond to changes in temperature and/or humidity. When you exercise, you probably breathe through your mouth. When this happens, cold, dry air gets into the lower airways without being warmed as it would be when breathing through the nose. Breathing through the nose can also help filter pollens, dirt, and molds. Outdoor exercise provides exposure to air-borne problems, and cold-weather sports mean more cold air is breathed in. Without being filtered through the nose, these allergens and cold air can cause problems.

Many believe swimming is an excellent sport for those with asthma. The warm, moist air at the surface of the pool provides a good environment. With proper treatment,

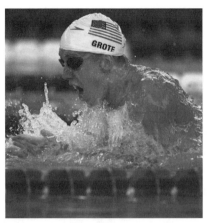

26 July 1996: Kurt Grote of the USA swims in the Men's 4 x 100 medley relay event in the 1996 Olympic Games at Georgia Tech Aquatic Center in Atlanta, Georgia.

Photo: David Cannon/Getty Images

Kurt Grote has had asthma all of his life. When he was younger, it often got in the way of exercise. He remembers being the last one picked for teams during gym class because classmates knew he would have to sit out most of the game or go to the nurse's office for treatments because he couldn't breathe. Things began to change for him in high school. He decided to try out the for school swim team. Although swimming wasn't easy at first and his coach even doubted his abilities, he stuck with the sport. He won a gold medal for the United States in 1996.

however, athletes excel in all sports, indoors and outdoors, in summer and in winter.

With proper medical advice, most teenagers with EIA can treat their asthma symptoms pre-exercise with a fast-acting inhaled medicine. Those with underlying asthma may also need to take daily, long-acting medications.

Sometimes athletes believe they can manage without medicine. This is a mistake. Managing your asthma symptoms with your doctor's help will not only make you a better athlete, it can also save your life.

It is best to be realistic about having asthma. It is better to avoid exercising in extremely cold weather, when you have a respiratory infection, when you are experiencing an increase in symptoms, or when pollen levels are high. Taking a break during those conditions doesn't make you a wimp. Using a fast-acting inhaler before you exercise doesn't make you a wimp either. Paying attention to your asthma symptoms makes you a mature, responsible person knowledgeable enough to take control. Whether you want to be a recreational athlete or a competitive athlete, learning what works best for your asthma symptoms will help you manage your exercise program in a way that lets you enjoy sports.

"I look at my asthma like the team I'm going to play against on Sunday," say professional football player Jerome Bettis, a member of the Asthma All-Star Program. "I train and I prepare to win."

Sometimes, however, despite pre-exercise treatments and even daily treatments, some teenagers can't participate in a particular sport. Perhaps the cold air of a winter sport produces problems despite your best efforts. In that case, look for a winter activity that takes place indoors— basketball, indoor track, gymnastics, or as mentioned earlier, indoor swimming. If you want to participate in athletics, there is a sport for you.

Sometimes sports that don't require continuous motion are the answer. Baseball, some track and field events, golf, or diving are some of the sports that allow for periods of inactivity during the game.

Maybe these changes in sport will mean you are a terrific swimmer instead of a football player, a competitive golfer instead of a field hockey player, or a record-setting high jumper instead of a soccer player. You *may* need to compromise to find the right sport for you. There are people with asthma in every sport, however. So, if your asthma symptoms are under control and you have made a plan with your doctor, get out there and give it a try.

Nocturnal (Nighttime) Asthma

It's the middle of the night. You wake up wheezing or coughing. Your chest feels tight. You felt fine during the day, but now at 2 A.M., you are having an asthma attack. What's going on?

If you have asthma, you have probably experienced a middle-of-the-night attack, but some people with asthma only experience nighttime episodes. These nighttime episodes are called nocturnal asthma. Although the symptoms show themselves at night, the condition exists all the time.

Body Rhythms

Specialists believe that nighttime symptoms may be related to our natural body rhythms called circadian rhythms. We naturally breathe best during the late afternoon hours and have our poorest breathing performance very early in the morning at about 4 A.M. During the late evening and early morning hours, the natural chemicals that are helpful in controlling asthma, epinephrine and cortisone, are at their lowest levels. If you have asthma, these fluctuations may create constrictions in your airways, provoking an asthma attack.

Sleeping Environment

Your sleeping environment may also play a role in provoking nighttime asthma attacks. For some, nighttime symptoms are provoked by allergies to substances in the bedroom—feather pillows, dust mites, and pet dander, for example. You can take steps to improve your sleeping environment. You can read more about this in chapter 4.

For those with sinus problems, the nighttime problems may be caused by chronic sinusitis or postnasal drip. A combination of treatments that helps control both asthma and sinus symptoms may reduce nighttime episodes.

Viral infections can also contribute to an increase in nighttime symptoms.

Heartburn

Although unusual in teenagers, many adults experience heartburn, or gastroesophageal reflux disease (GERD). Stomach acids make their way into the esophagus and throat and irritate the bronchial tubes. Symptoms of gastric reflux are greater at night and may provoke nighttime asthma attacks. Treating the heartburn may help improve the asthma.

Performance Problems

Frequent nighttime attacks also affect performance. You may think that nighttime episodes only affect you at night.

However, if you are waking at night with asthma episodes, you are not getting enough sleep. You may feel exhausted most of the time. Your school work may suffer and your athletic performance may suffer, too. Those who have asthma attacks at night are more likely to miss school.

Although you may not have trouble during the day, nighttime symptoms mean your asthma is *not* under control. As the asthma classification chart shows, increases in nighttime symptoms are one of the measures used to rate the severity of your asthma. Those with mild intermittent asthma have nighttime symptoms infrequently while those with severe persistent asthma are often affected by nighttime episodes. Nighttime symptoms should be taken seriously as a fatal asthma attack is more likely to happen at night. (Read more about this in chapter 7.) If you are experiencing asthma symptoms at night, your doctor can help you develop a treatment plan to better manage your symptoms.

Cough-Variant (Hidden) Asthma

Hack, hack, hack. Cough-variant asthma presents itself as the cough that just won't go away. Often those with this type of asthma have few other symptoms—no wheezing or shortness of breath. This type of asthma is often identified after all other suspected causes have been eliminated.

Occupational Asthma

Doctors recognized an association between asthma symptoms and jobs as far back as the early 1700s when Bernardino Ramazzini, an Italian physician, described a link between certain patients' asthma and their specific occupations. He recognized even then that bakers exposed to wheat and rye flour, mill workers exposed to grain dust, and farmers sensitive to animal dander were affected by their jobs.

Today, asthma caused by exposure to an irritant at work is called occupational asthma. The Occupational Safety and

RISKY JOBS

- Animal handlers
- Bakers
- Cleaning and janitorial workers
- Detergent manufacturers
- Farming and agricultural workers
- Health care workers
- Jewelry makers
- Lab workers
- Nickel platers
- Snow crab and egg processors
- Solderers
- Workers with paint, plastics, adhesives, grains, red cedar, metal salts

❖ Up to 30 percent of all bakers are affected by occupational asthma.
❖ 17 percent of health care workers develop allergic reactions to latex gloves.

Health Administration of the United States Department of Labor (OSHA) estimates that 11 million workers are exposed to one of the more than 200 agents associated with the development of occupational asthma. OSHA estimates that 15 percent of the disabling asthma cases in the United States are job related.

There are two types of occupational asthma. One develops after a period of "sensitization" to an agent in the workplace. This is called immunologic asthma. Many health care workers develop allergies to latex following exposure to latex gloves.

Irritant-induced asthma occurs after exposure to an irritating dust, mist, vapor, or fume. Bakers have the highest incidence of occupational asthma because they are exposed to high levels of flour dust.

If your asthma symptoms develop or worsen after taking a new job, if you feel better when you are away from work (especially during longer periods away like weekends or vacations), if you asthma symptoms worsen during the time you are at work, speak to your doctor. Your job could be making you sick. According to the NHLBI, "ideal management" of occupational asthma requires complete avoidance of the trigger as continued exposure can lead to increasingly severe and potentially fatal asthma attacks. You may have to leave your job to avoid the triggers or you may need to move to a different department away from the irritating triggers. Even after you have been away from the trigger, job-related asthma symptoms can continue for up to two years.

For some, a personal respirator might be the answer.

Sinus-Related Asthma

Many teenagers with sinus problems also have asthma. When nasal passages are inflamed, doctors call this condition rhinitis. Symptoms of rhinitis might include post-nasal drip, congestion, a runny nose, and/or sneezing. When the nasal cavities surrounding the nose and near the cheekbones and eyes become blocked, normal secretions cannot flow and may collect bacteria. This bacteria is the cause of sinus infections. Sometimes people with sinus problems are unaware of the condition, but if you have sinus problems, it is likely you experience headaches (some describe the pain as a "face ache"). The area under and around your eyes may be sensitive to pressure, your nose may feel stuffy, and your ears may feel plugged. Many people with sinus problems also have asthma. Doctors aren't sure exactly what complicates the relationship, but many suspect that misinformation may play a part. Somehow the brain confuses the messages the sinuses send out and believes the messages are coming from the lungs. The brain then sends a message to the lungs causing them to respond with swelling and inflammation. Often treating rhinitis and sinusitis reduces asthma symptoms.

Aspirin-Induced Asthma (AIA)

Some asthmatics are sensitive to aspirin and other nonsteroid anti-inflammatory drugs. Although aspirin-induced asthma is rare in children, it may occur in teenagers. Few young people take aspirin as it is associated with Reye's Syndrome, but many adults use aspirin. Up to 50 percent of adults with severe asthma have AIA, 30 percent of those with moderate asthma, and 20 percent of those with mild asthma. Those who have sinus problems, rhinitis, or nasal polyps are at greater risk. Respiratory infections seem to be involved in the development of aspirin sensitivity.

In general, a reaction to asthma follows within an hour of taking aspirin. Flushing, eye irritation, and nasal congestion can precede or occur along with asthma symptoms. This type of allergy is very serious and can lead to death.

Steroid-Resistant Asthma

For most people with asthma, treatments with steroid drugs called corticosteroids or glucocorticoids reduce airway inflammation, helping them to breathe. You can read more about this in chapter 5. For some people, however, treatment with this type of medicine is not effective. Sometimes this type of asthma is called *difficult* asthma or steroid-resistant asthma because it doesn't respond to traditional treatments.

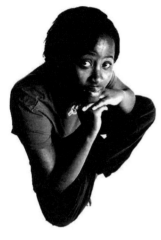

Although only a small percentage of people with asthma have steroid-resistant asthma, the number of sufferers is estimated at about 750,000 people. Researchers have found that African American patients are more resistant to the anti-inflammatory drugs most often used to treat asthma. If you are an African American teenager, these statistics may be especially troublesome. Black teenagers are three times more likely than white teenagers to have steroid-resistant asthma. Researchers suspect African Americans with asthma have more severe inflammation, making treatment more difficult, or that they may have a genetic resistance to the drug.

Doctors diagnose steroid-resistant asthma when a patient does not improve at least 15 percent following a two-week treatment with oral prednisone, a steroid drug.

You can read more about avoiding triggers for asthma in the next chapter and more about asthma treatment in chapter 5.

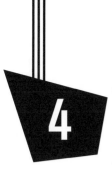

4

Asthma Triggers and How to Avoid Them

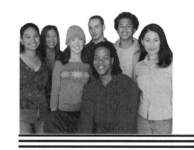

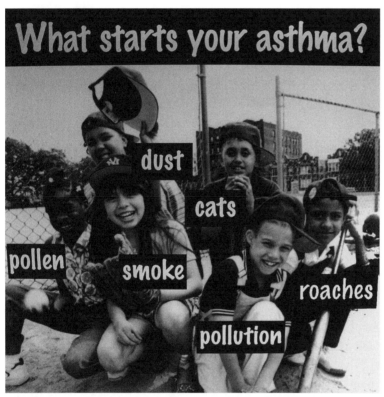

As this poster shows, not everyone is affected by the same asthma triggers. This poster was developed by the New York City Department of Health and Mental Hygiene. Stuart Pittman, design. Michael Paras, photography.

As you read in the previous chapters, asthma is a chronic condition. Sometimes you experience symptoms of the condition—you wheeze, you are short of breath, you feel tired, or you experience uncontrollable coughing. Sometimes, however, you don't feel those symptoms. That doesn't mean your asthma is cured. It simply means your asthma is under control.

If you have asthma, your airways are hypersensitive. When they are irritated, they respond with swelling, tightening, and by producing excess mucus. Doctors call the substances that cause these irritations triggers. As asthma is different in every person, the triggers that can make asthma symptoms worse vary from person to person. One of the best ways of helping to keep your asthma under control is to avoid exposure to the triggers that are problems for you.

INDOOR TRIGGERS

Dust

A significant culprit in the trigger department is dust. Perhaps you, like many teens with asthma, are sensitive to dust. Dust is made up of many particles including fibers, mold, pollen, insects and insect feces, animal danders, and dust mites and mite feces. Most often it is the dust mites within the dust that create the problem. Dust mites are eight-legged creatures that are so small that you can't see them. Thousands of these arthropods can live on one dust particle. Their bodies, secretions, and feces are the main source of dust allergens that can make asthma worse. They thrive on the microscopic dander or skin flakes that we shed each day and flourish in areas where we sleep. They love mattresses, pillows, and comforters. According to the American Medical Association, more than 2 million dust mites can set up housekeeping in one mattress. Unfortunately, they live on those stuffed animals many of us like to snuggle with each night, too. Dust mites can live on carpeting, upholstered furniture, in draperies, and in air ducts as well. Because so many people are sensitive to dust mites, doctors recommend attacking the bedroom in an effort to reduce exposure to the tiny creatures and

> **More than two million dust mites can live on one mattress!**

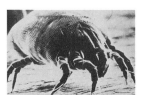

Dust mite

Image provided by the American Academy of Allergy, Asthma and Immunology

their droppings. Many companies sell special coverings to help dustproof mattresses, box springs, and pillows. Ask your doctor for the name of a local store that carries allergy supplies. All bedding should be washable. Although those cozy feather comforters must go, those wonderfully soft washable fleece blankets make comfy replacements. Someone in your family should wash your sheets and blankets in very hot water once a week and give your furry, stuffed friends a ride in the washing machine, too. If you have rugs on your floor, you might want to have your parents remove them from your room. By the time you are a teen, cleaning your room should be your job, but if you are allergic to dust mites, it is probably best if someone else does the cleaning. Dust particles get airborne in the process and it is a good idea for you to be out of the room while cleaning takes place. If someone else has to clean your room, you should take on cleaning responsibilities that don't provoke your asthma symptoms. Maybe you could take care of the dishes and the trash, and your sibling can change beds, dust, or vacuum.

A thorough cleaning will produce the best results. According to the National Institute of Allergy and Infectious Diseases's (NIAID) *How to Create a Dust-Free Bedroom* fact sheet, cleaning will not only help remove dust mites, but insect dust as well. They make the following suggestions:

- **Completely empty the room.**
- **Empty, clean, and seal all closets or keep clothing in zippered plastic bags and shoes in boxes off the floor.**
- **Remove carpeting, if possible.**
- **Clean and scrub the woodwork and floors thoroughly to remove all traces of dust.**
- **Wipe wood, tile, or linoleum floors with water, wax, or oil.**
- **If you have linoleum, cement it to the floor.**
- **Close the doors and windows until the dust-sensitive person is ready to occupy the room.**

When vacuuming, vacuums with HEPA filters and double-thickness bags are best. Reducing the humidity in your room will also help. Dehumidifiers or air conditioners can help.

ROACH FACTS

Did You Know?

▶ Roaches have blood that is almost white and they can breathe through their sides.

▶ Roaches have been around since before the dinosaurs.

▶ Roaches can swim. A roach can hold its breath for 40 minutes!

▶ Most roaches live in tropical places like rain forests. Even though there are several thousand different kinds, only about five are commonly found in people's homes.

For more information about roaches and pest control, visit the interactive EPA Web site, Help It's a Roach, www.epa.gov/pesticides/kids/roaches/english/facts/index.html

Cockroaches

As if dust mites aren't disgusting enough, another multilegged creature also causes serious asthma problems, cockroaches! Once again, not only the creature, but its droppings are responsible for increased asthma symptoms. Cockroaches are hard to get rid of. They have been around for more than 300 million years and will probably be around for that many more. Roach dust contains microscopic roach body parts and roach droppings that provoke asthma symptoms in many people. Roach dust can make asthma attacks more frequent and more serious. Those who live in urban areas where roach populations are often large are the most at risk. A recent study by the National Institute of Allergy and Infectious Disease (NIAID) found that 37 percent of inner-city children tested were allergic to cockroaches. The allergy combined with the high levels of cockroach allergen levels placed those children at risk for more serious asthma problems. They were hospitalized more often, they missed school more often, they needed nearly twice as many unscheduled asthma-related medical visits, and suffered more often from asthma-related loss of sleep. These studies may help explain why illness and death from asthma are particularly high among urban African Americans.

According to NIAID director Dr. Anthony S. Fauci, "some of the most vulnerable of our citizens, children in the poorest neighborhoods of our largest cities, suffer disproportionately from asthma."

So, what can you do about it? Don't feed the animals! You can keep those snacks out of the area where you spend most of your time—your bedroom. If you go into the kitchen for a snack, put food back into covered containers or into the refrigerator when you are finished making your snack. Wash your dishes and wipe off the counter after you are finished. If you can't wash dishes right away, put them in a sink with soapy water (roaches can't live in soapy water). Clean up your pets' food dishes, too. Put them away at night. Keep trash in a container with lid and take the trash out every day. Try to remove any food source that attracts insects.

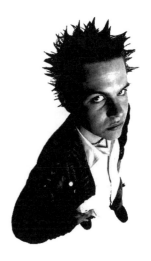

If you can't starve the little buggers, let them die of thirst. Don't leave any standing liquids—no half-full bottles of cola, no partially consumed glass of water, no water left in the sink or the tub. Your parents should look for any water leaks in sinks or washing machines, or leaks on walls or on the roof. Even the drip pan of the refrigerator can provide water for insects.

You can try to keep roaches out of your home. They love clutter—old newspapers, stacks of grocery bags, etc. Clutter gives them a cozy place to hide. Spray foam, mesh wire, and even copper wool pads can be used to block holes in the wall to help keep roaches out.

What you shouldn't do is try to kill them with roach sprays, fogger, or bombs. They aren't effective and may make your asthma symptoms worse. If necessary, your parents may need to try insect control substances like poison baits, traps, or gels. The Environmental Health Watch of Cleveland has produced an online Cockroach Control Guide at www.ehw.org/Asthma/ASTH_Cockroach_Control.htm. If you have access to a computer, you can download their recommendations and give them to your mom or dad. They recommend using bait gels or stations to combat roaches. Insects eat the bait food, go back into hiding, and die. When other roaches eat the dead roach, they die, too. Of course, these baits must be placed out of the reach of children and pets. Roaches are pretty smart. They won't eat from bait sources if bug sprays or harsh chemicals have been used nearby.

If you live in an apartment, your landlord is probably responsible for helping control roaches. Cooperate with control policies by controlling the factors that increase roach populations within your apartment.

Unfortunately, getting rid of the pests is not enough. Body parts and droppings can linger in house dust for a long time and continue to trigger asthma symptoms. Surfaces need to be cleaned, and bleach can help kill the chemicals in roach dust that provoke asthma symptoms.

Rodent droppings and urine are common asthma triggers, especially in urban environments.

However, many people with asthma are sensitive to the smell of bleach. You should not be around when cleaning takes place. Rugs should be vacuumed with a special vacuum with a HEPA filter, if possible. If your family doesn't have this type of vacuum, use a vacuum that is already partly filled. Less dust is released into the air than when an empty bag is used. If carpets can be washed, wash them.

It may be necessary to remove carpeting. Again, anyone with asthma should not be present when carpets are removed, and the room should be sealed. The carpet should be removed in sections, wrapped in plastic, and sealed. The floor should be mopped as each section is removed.

Rodents

Rats! More varmints. Keeping rodents as pets is not a good idea if you have asthma. Most of us who come into contact with mice or rats, however, don't do it intentionally. Rats and mice live in all neighborhoods, but they live in higher numbers where, like roaches, they can find food and water. This is why they are more of a problem in urban areas. Recent findings indicate that rodent droppings and urine are common triggers of asthma symptoms. Researchers used information gathered from the 1996

National Cooperative Inner-City Asthma Study and found that mice played a significant role as an asthma trigger. They examined the homes of 608 inner-city children with asthma. They discovered that a whopping 95 percent of the homes had detectable mouse allergen in at least one room. Eighty-seven percent of the kitchens, bedrooms, and living rooms had detectable mouse urine or dander. Doctors then skin tested 499 of those children and discovered that 18 percent were allergic to mouse allergen. This combination of high levels of allergen and sensitivity to mouse allergen lead to increased symptoms for the young people. Lead investigator, Dr. Robert Wood, associate professor of pediatrics at Johns Hopkins said, "Mouse (allergens) appear to be more of a factor than things like dust mites or cats and dogs that we've traditionally thought of as being the most important indoor allergens. So, in the inner-city environment, we would still have cockroach number one, but mouse is probably in second place and ahead of things like dust mites." He recommends aggressive extermination of both mice and cockroaches.

Again, you can help keep the rodent population down by adapting the same strategies used for controlling roaches. In addition to restricting food and water sources and closing up holes in walls, some further precautions may be needed. Rats and mice can gnaw right through plastic garbage bags. Keep garbage in heavy plastic or metal containers with lids. Keep foods in metal or glass containers with tight lids. If you have a pet, store its food in a closed container as well. Bags of cat food, dog food, and bird food are easy pickings for rodents. If your pet spends time outside, clean up its eating area and clean up its droppings. It may be hard to believe, but dog excrement actually attracts rats. Clean up around your house. Get rid of tall grass and any trash in the area. Clean up places where rodents can hide. If, despite your best efforts, you are still having problems with rodents, your city or town may have a rodent control program. Your parents can call your local Board of Health. They may also need to call a professional certified exterminator. Rodents carry many diseases, and if

you have asthma and are sensitive to rodent urine or
dander, you have even more reason to get rid of them. It is
a sensible step in helping control another asthma trigger.

Pets

Many people with asthma are allergic to animals.
Flakes of the animal's skin, or dander, and dried saliva can
cause problems for people with asthma—sometimes severe
problems. Up to 50 percent of young people with asthma
are triggered by an allergy to cats or dogs. Most are
allergic to cats. Some are allergic to birds. The urine from
rodents (guinea pigs, rats, rabbits, and gerbils) can cause
problems, too.

There is probably nothing more difficult for young
people than having to deal with a pet allergy. Unfortunately,
the best thing to do about it is to keep the animal out of
your home. It is hard if that means you can't get a cat, a
dog, or a gerbil, but it is especially painful if you already
have a pet. For some, the only option is to give the animal
to a loving home. Before giving up your pet, however, be

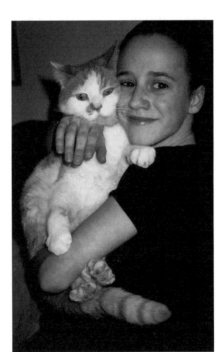

Ashley

**Ashley had her first asthma
attack following a
respiratory infection.
Fortunately, she isn't
allergic to cats.**

Photo: R. Anthony Silva

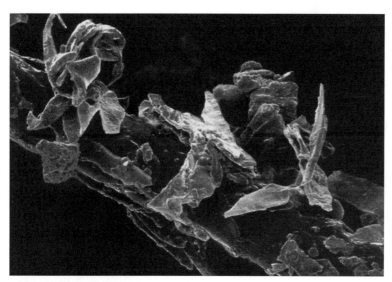

Animal dander

Animal dander image provided by the American Academy of Allergy, Asthma and Immunology

sure the animal is causing your problems. An allergist can give you a test to determine if you are allergic to animals.

According to Dr. Wood, "A diagnosis of cat or dog allergy can be made by a skin test or blood test. If the test is negative, it is very unlikely that cat or dog exposure will affect asthma in any way. However, if the test is positive, then it is very likely that animal exposure will lead to worsening of asthma. . . ." (Read more about allergy testing in chapter 3.)

If it is necessary to remove a pet from your home, you can expect to feel sad, but don't expect your asthma symptoms to get better immediately after your pet leaves. Allergen levels fall slowly. It can take as long as six months before lingering cat allergens are gone. In the long run, however, limiting your exposure to an animal you are allergic to will improve your symptoms, reduce the amount of medicine you need to take, and in general improve the way you feel. It is hard and it may be hard to accept, but *you* are more important than your pet.

Sometimes allergies are less serious and taking measures to avoid the animal dander can help limit your exposure. No matter how much you enjoy having your pet curl up on your bed, animals should *not* sleep in your bedroom. In fact, they shouldn't go into your bedroom at all, so keep your bedroom door closed. Keep the air vents in your room covered. Try to keep your pet in one room of the house. We all know how much cats and dogs love to get up on the furniture. Try to keep them off upholstered pieces. Their fur collects there. While washing your pet (even cats) can help reduce allergens in the air, Dr. Wood says the benefits of the washings are short lived and may not be worth the trouble.

There is some promising news for those who love cats. Dr. David Avner is in the process of developing allergen-free cats. His company Transgenic Pets is working to eliminate the gene in cats responsible for causing allergic reactions in humans. Dr. Avner expects the first allergen-free cats to be available next year. To follow his progress, visit www.transgenicpets.com.

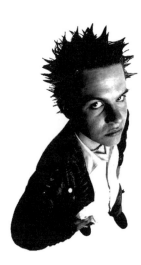

Mold and Mildew

The fungus is among us. According to *The World Book Encyclopedia*, the word mildew comes from the Middle English word *mealdew,* which means spoiled meal. While there are two types of mildew, powdery mildew and downy mildew (which damage living plants), the terms is generally used to describe any fungus that grows in damp areas.

Molds, sometimes called mildew, are parasitic, microscopic fungi that need water to survive. Molds are found indoors and outdoors and can be asthma triggers for some people.

Indoors, mold presents a special challenge. Molds can enter our homes in the air, on insects, on pets, or on our clothing. While reproducing, molds release spores that land on wet or damp surfaces and begin growing and multiplying. Inhaling or touching these spores can trigger asthma symptoms in those allergic to mold. These fungi can cause allergic reactions including runny nose, eye irritation, cough, congestion, and most importantly for you, an increase in asthma symptoms.

Experts aren't sure why mold spores trigger asthma symptoms. It may be that they are so tiny that they can easily enter and irritate the respiratory system. It may be that the mold contains a protein that some people are allergic to. Perhaps the chemicals that mold produces irritate the respiratory system. Although the exact cause of the response is uncertain, the results of mold exposure in sensitive people is not. Depending on the severity of your allergy, it may take only a few mold spores to provoke symptoms or it may take significant mold contamination to trigger your asthma.

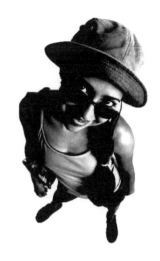

Molds cannot grow without moisture. They thrive in dark, damp, humid areas like basements, bathrooms, and attics. They love dirty places like garbage containers and clean places like clothes dryers. They like cool places like air conditioners and refrigerators, and warm places like shower stalls. They grow inside of books, newspapers, and magazines. Any spot that is damp will make a nice place for mold to grow. Sometimes we can see the mold on showers, growing on walls, or on other surfaces in basements. If damp clothes are left on the floor or in a laundry basket for more than a day or two, you may see it growing on them. It may look black, green, or red.

Sometimes the only way we know mold is a problem is when we smell it. That damp, musty spell is caused by chemical changes taking place as the mold produces waste products. The smell is a sign that mold is growing and needs attention.

Fortunately, mold cannot grow without moisture, so the best way to control mold is to limit moisture in your home. Although it is impossible to keep mold spores outside the home, it is possible to prevent them from thriving. Once mold gets established, it is difficult to remove (see below). The best course is to prevent it from growing in the first place.

Because the bathroom is such a moist, warm place, it is often the first place mold grows in a home. You can help prevent mold growth by running a fan or leaving a window open while you shower. That will help prevent moisture buildup in the room. Wipe down the shower walls when you are finished showering. Don't leave your damp towel in a heap where there will be little air circulation on the wet material. Instead, hang it up. Don't throw wet towels or clothes onto the floor or into the clothes hamper either. If they remain there for more than a day, mold may begin to grow on them. If your clothes are damp, hang them up and let them dry before putting them in the hamper. Don't put wet shoes inside a closet or inside a gym bag. Leave them out in the air (preferably outside) to dry.

Have your parents or your landlord look for any leaks in the bathroom and repair them.

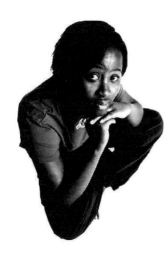

Kitchens are another place where damp items can attract mold. Discard out-of-date food before mold begins to grow. Wipe down and dry surfaces in the refrigerator and change the drip pan regularly. Wipe up spills as soon as they happen. You can reduce the humidity in the kitchen by keeping pots covered while cooking and by running a kitchen exhaust fan if one is available. If you have plants inside your home, the moisture they need to survive may be the same moisture the mold needs to flourish. If you are having a problem with mold, you may need to remove plants from inside your home.

Leaks in walls or roofs can allow moisture into your home. If you see wet areas or smell musty odors on walls, make sure your parents are aware of the problem. In case of water damage, repairs and cleanup should begin immediately to prevent mold growth. Run a dehumidifier or air conditioner. Humidity levels below 60 percent will inhibit mold growth.

Unfortunately, mold can hide in places we can't see. It can grow in ceiling tiles, behind sheet rock, beneath carpets, and inside heating ducts. If there is serious mold growth in your home or if you have experienced flooding in your home you should stay away while a qualified professional cleans and/or removes any moldy items. If your parents choose to try to do the cleanup themselves, they should consult the Environmental Protection Agency's (EPA) website for recommendations (www.epa.gov/iag/molds/moldguide.html) and wear an approved respirator, rubber gloves, and protective goggles. The first step in any cleanup process has to be eliminating the source of moisture. If faucets or drains are leaking, they must be repaired. If there are cracks in walls that allow moisture to enter, they must be sealed. No cleanup process will work if the source of the water is not addressed.

Bleach solutions or fungicides are sometimes used during mold cleanup. That can present problems if you are sensitive to the fumes. Your parents should be sure windows are open to allow for ventilation, and again, you should stay away during cleaning. It is not sufficient to simply spray moldy areas with a cleaning product. According to North Carolina's Department of Health, these solutions may kill the mold, but they will not eliminate the problem. Even dead mold particles when airborne can present health risks if you are sensitive to mold.

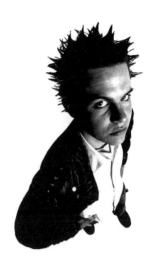

In general, nonporous items can be cleaned and dried—tile, glass, hard plastic, etc. Semiporous items like wood, plaster, and concrete can usually be cleaned. However, porous items like carpeting, sheetrock, wallpaper, fabric, upholstered furniture, and carpeting will need to be removed from your home. Moldy items removed from your home should be wrapped in plastic and sealed.

If you see mold in your home and suspect it is contributing to your asthma symptoms, talk to your parents.

Tobacco Smoke

One of the most problematic triggers for asthmatics is cigarette smoke. Cigarette smoking is dangerous for anyone, but for asthmatics smoking worsens asthma symptoms. If you are a smoker, even an occasional smoker, try to stop now. According to the 1999 National Youth Tobacco Survey, the number of cigarettes young smokers consume increases with age. While you may only smoke one or two cigarettes a day in your early teen years, smoking is addictive and you can expect to be smoking much more each year. The average teen smoker begins smoking at about 12 years old. By the

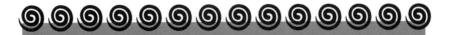

RESOURCES TO HELP YOU QUIT SMOKING

American Lung Association
Freedom from Smoking Online
www.lungusa.org/ffs/

CDC's You Can Quit Smoking Guide
www.cdc.gov/tobacco/quit/canquit.htm

Health A-Z.com

Ways to Kick the Habit
www.healthatoz.com (key words: Kick the Habit)

How Can I Quit Smoking
kidshealth.org/teen/drug_alcohol/tobacco/quit_smoking.html

QuitNet
www.quitnet.com/

Quit4Life
www.quit4life.com
A look at how four young people were able to quit smoking.

Quitting Smoking
American Lung Association
www.lungusa.org/tobacco/quitting_smoke.html

21 Secrets of Successful Quitters
NicotineFreeKids
www.nicotinefreekids.com

The Whole Truth Campaign
Florida Department of Health
Division of Health Awareness and Tobacco
4025 Esplanade Way
Tallahassee, FL 32399-1743
(850) 245-4144
www.gen-swat.com

time you reach high school, you may find yourself among the 16.7 percent of students who describe themselves as frequent smokers. Most young smokers want to quit and most believe they can. Unfortunately, most are not successful. If you want some strong motivation to stop, visit www.gen-swat.com and discover how cigarette manufacturers are manipulating you.

According to the Global Initiatives for Asthma report from the National Institutes of Health, "active smoking is associated with accelerated decline of lung function in people with asthma, greater asthma severity, and poor response to asthma treatment. . . ."

If you don't smoke, you may still be seriously affected by cigarette smoke. For asthmatics, second-hand smoke is a dangerous trigger. Children who grow up in homes with smokers are more likely to develop asthma. Those who live with smokers experience more severe asthma symptoms. Unfortunately, this affects up to 1 million young people. If you live with smokers, tell them that smoking makes your asthma worse. Often they are unaware of the effects their smoking can have on an asthmatic's condition. Encourage them to stop smoking, or if they are unable to stop, to smoke outside of the house.

Nancy Sandler's *A Parents Guide to Asthma* gives excellent encouragement for parents who are having difficulty with smoking. She compares the irritation in an asthmatic's lung with a skinned knee. The surface is sensitive and raw. Parents would never pour irritating chemicals on a skinned knee, says she. Why then would they want to fill irritated lungs with chemicals by smoking? If you find it difficult to ask your parents or siblings not to smoke around you, ask your doctor to speak to them. Some young people feel so strongly about living with smokers that they have gone to court to have their parents stop smoking around them. Most recently, the mother of a 13-year-old boy was banned from smoking in her house and in her car after her son complained that he didn't want to visit his mother because she smoked.

> Recently, the mother of a thirteen-year-old boy was banned from smoking in her house and car.

Teens often have no trouble telling their parents what to do, but they have much more difficulty telling their friends. If your friends smoke, let them know that smoking around you is a problem. Give them the example Nancy Sandler uses. Would they pour turpentine on a cut? If they are your friends, they will limit their smoking. You will be doing them a favor, too, because they won't be smoking as often.

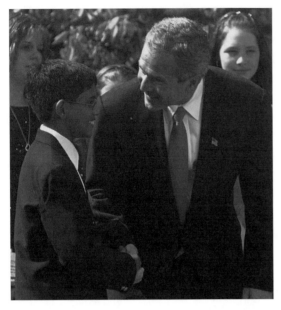

Amit Bushan and President George W. Bush

White House photo by Paul Morse

Amit Bushan of Lubbock, Texas, was one of thirty winners of the President's Environmental Youth Awards. He launched the "Stop Tobacco in Restaurants" (STIR) campaign in his hometown. His work led to a local ordinance banning smoking in all public places. He received his award from President Bush in the White House Rose Garden on April 18, 2002.

Amit's work was inspired by his asthma. Unable to enjoy one of his favorite sports, bowling, because his local bowling alley allowed smoking, and unable to linger over a restaurant meal because smoke there aggravated his asthma, he decided to do something about it. He initiated his work with a presentation at his school, highlighting the harmful effects of second-hand smoke.

With the encouragement of his school principal and with the help of several friends, he began a letter-writing campaign and presented the letters at a meeting of the Lubbock City Council. The council formed a group to study the problem and they agreed that second-hand smoke is a health hazard.

In October 2001, smoking was banned in all but a few public places in Lubbock. Bars, sports grills, and bingo parlors were exempted from the legislation. Businesses have three years to comply with the ordinance, so pretty soon Amit will be able to go bowling again.

In addition to bowling, Amit likes to play basketball, spend time with his friends, and swim for the Lubbock Swim Club. He has had asthma since he was five.

Illegal Drugs

A small, but not insignificant number of acute and life threatening asthma attacks may be triggered by heroin inhalation. Although no formal studies have been completed, doctors in one Chicago hospital reported that between 1998 and 2000, one-third to one-half of their asthma patients under age fifty may have had some link with inhaled heroin. They reported that the problem is not confined to inner cities. Adults and teenagers are using increasingly pure forms of heroin and putting their lives at risk not only from the drug itself, but from asthma complications associated with the inhaled form. To date, doctors are unsure if the heroin itself causes the breathing problems, if it contains an irritant in the powder used to cut the drug, or if heroin users neglect treatment for their asthma and ignore the warning signs of acute attacks.

Indoor Air Pollution

In addition to cigarettes, wood-burning stoves, gas stoves, heaters, clothes dryers, kerosene heaters, and fireplaces can emit fumes that provoke asthma symptoms in some people. The EPA calls the emissions from these items "combustion pollutants." They are gases or particles that come from burning materials. Natural gas, liquid propane gas, fuel oil, kerosene, wood, and coal can produce indoor air pollution. The levels of pollution depend on the type of appliance being used; how well it is installed, maintained, and vented; and the kind of fuel it uses. These fuels produce pollutants including carbon monoxide, nitrogen dioxide, particles, and sulfur dioxide. Some appliances also produce unburned hydrocarbons and aldehydes. While these indoor pollutants are not good for anyone, they are especially harmful to sensitive individuals including asthmatics.

Breathing high levels of nitrogen dioxide can irritate the respiratory system. If you have asthma, you are probably more susceptible to the effects of nitrogen dioxide. Sulfur dioxide can also irritate the airways. Exposure to sulfur dioxide can cause wheezing, chest tightness, or breathing problems especially in those with asthma. Particle matter that is released when fuels are not completely burned can also irritate the lungs.

Several studies have shown a higher incidence of asthma hospitalizations in asthmatic individuals who cook with gas. Poorly vented heating, drying, and cooking appliances can also release fumes that aggravate asthma symptoms. According to Pat Musto, a nurse writing for the *Allergy and Asthma Advocate*, indoor pollutants including wood-burning stoves can provoke breathing problems. Poorly vented woodstoves and the use of "poorly combustible and gas-emitting products (treated and pressed wood, garbage, uncured wood) are particularly hazardous. Fireplaces and woodstoves should be properly vented to decrease indoor pollutants.

The EPA gives the following advice to help reduce exposure to indoor pollutants:

◎ **Fuel-Burning, Unvented Heaters**
When using a space heater, your parents should follow the manufacturer's directions, making sure the flame is properly adjusted. A yellow-tipped flame is an indication that the heater needs to be adjusted. You can help with ventilation by opening a door from the room where the heater is located to the rest of the house and opening a window.

◎ **Gas Stoves and Fireplaces**
Use a stove hood with a fan vented to the outside to reduce exposure to pollutants. Again, a yellow-tipped flame is a sign of pollutant emissions. Have your parents call the gas company to adjust the burner so the tip of the flame is blue. If your parents are shopping for a new stove, encourage them to consider an electric stove or at least a gas stove without a pilot light that burns continually. Newer stoves have electric ignition systems. If you have a gas-burning fireplace, be sure the flue is open when in use.

◎ **Woodstoves**
Again, your parents need to follow the manufacturer's directions for using the woodstove. The door to the woodstove should fit snuggly. Burn aged or cured wood. Never burn pressure-treated wood. It contains dangerous chemicals. When adding wood, open the stove's damper. This allows more air to circulate and keeps the smoke from going into your house and allows it to move up the chimney and out of the house.

◎ **Furnaces, Chimneys, and Flues**
Furnaces, chimneys, and flues must be maintained. If they are blocked, leaking, or damaged they can release harmful gases and particles, and even dangerous levels of carbon dioxide. Your parents will need to change the filters according to the manufacturer's recommendations.

For more information, consult the EPA guide, *The Inside Story: A Guide to Indoor Air Quality*" at www.epa.gov/iaq/pubs/insidest.html.

Other Inhaled Irritants

Does your mother's hairspray make you wheeze? Does the smell of your sister's talcum powder make you short of breath? Does your brother's aftershave make you cough? Although marketers and manufacturers are convinced we love the smell of these colognes, sprays, lotions, powders, and soaps, for those with asthma, a whiff of these products can be enough to make us wheeze, cough, and choke. Cosmetics, body lotions, deodorants, aerosol sprays, soap, shampoos, and conditioners can all trigger asthma symptoms. Most beauty products now come in unscented versions. If you are sensitive to the smell of these products, ask your family members to switch to unscented varieties.

In addition to these beauty products, a host of indoor beautification products can cause asthma symptoms as well. Many people with asthma are sensitive to the smell of cleaning products, air fresheners, potpourri, garden chemicals, mothballs, detergents, fabric softeners, glues, and/or paints. If you have asthma and are sensitive to these smells, it is best that you leave the house while cleaning and painting are going on. Maybe you could arrange to spend the night with your grandparents, your cousins, or with one of your friends when major home projects are going on.

Food

Many young people with food allergies develop asthma. Recent studies indicate that food can trigger asthma symptoms in 6 to 8 percent of young people with asthma. Foods that are most often identified as problems are milk, eggs, peanuts, tree nuts, soy, wheat, fish, and crustaceans. Some cheeses contain mold that can act as an asthma trigger. Although many children outgrow food allergies by the time they are three or four, many teens continue to be allergic to peanuts, tree nuts, or shellfish. Unfortunately, the numbers of life-threatening and fatal incidents related to foods have increased significantly over the past twenty years, and teens seem to be especially vulnerable. This may be because teens eat away from home more often than younger children.

Although these teens know about their food allergies, they may eat the life-threatening food without being aware of it.

Sometimes the foods are hidden ingredients in restaurant dishes. Who would think chili might have peanuts in it? How many people know that pesto sauce is made with nuts? It is the hidden ingredient that causes most of the problems. Young people with allegies know not to order the chicken in peanut sauce, the shrimp tempura, or the peanut butter sandwich. It is what they don't know that gets them into trouble. Unfortunately, asking the waiter or waitress about food ingredients can be dangerous. Only the chef or cook knows what actually goes into the restaurant food. If you know you have a food allergy and want to eat in restaurants, address your ingredients questions to the people who actually prepare the food.

Because food allergies can be life threatening, anyone with food allergies should take serious precautions to avoid specific foods and food additives (see below). Unfortunately, so many processed foods include ingredients we would never suspect as part of the food, and sometimes food labels are inaccurate. To protect yourself, you should work closely with your doctor to develop an emergency plan.

Always carry an inhaler. Your doctor may also prescribe an EpiPen, an automatic epinephrine injection system that is shaped like a pen. When pressed against the body (usually the outer thigh), the pen automatically injects a premeasured amount of epinephrine. If your doctor prescribes one for you, be sure to carry it with you. It may save your life. Your doctor might also recommend an antihistamine like Benadryl.

EpiPens deliver a premeasured amount of epinephrine. EpiPens saves lives.

Not only do you need to carry your medicines, but you also need to be ready to use them at the first sign of trouble. An itchy mouth, hives, tingling, flushing, itching, wheezing, abdominal cramps, and/or vomiting may be the first signs of an allergic reaction. Don't wait to see if the symptoms get better or go away. Sometimes the symptoms may disappear only to come back more violently later. In a recent study of near-fatal and fatal food exposures, all those who survived received epinephrine within five minutes of experiencing symptoms.

If you think certain foods may be triggering your asthma symptoms, you should discuss food allergy testing with your doctor.

Food Additives

In addition to allergies to specific foods, two food additives, monosodium glutamate (MSG) and sulfites, can present problems for a small number of people with asthma. MSG is a food flavor enhancer and is used in packaged foods, foods prepared in restaurants, and foods prepared at home. While most people (even asthmatics) can eat MSG without adverse reactions, most doctors believed that asthmatics who are also sensitive to MSG may have negative reactions to the additive including bronchospasm. However, two recent studies indicate that MSG may not be an important asthma trigger. Research continues in this area. Talk to your doctor if you believe you are sensitive to MSG.

The Food and Drug Administration (FDA) estimates that about 1 percent of the general population is sensitive to sulfites and that about 5 percent of asthmatics are sulfite sensitive. Those who have severe asthma symptoms and are dependent on corticosteroids (see the next chapter) are at greatest risk of having a severe reaction. According to the FDA, among items containing sulfites are drinks including beer, wine, hard cider, fruit and vegetable juices, and tea; and a variety of cooked and processed foods including baked goods, condiments (pickled foods), dried fruits, jam, gravy, dehydrated or precut or peeled fresh potatoes, molasses, shrimp, soup mixes, canned vegetables, maraschino cherries, and guacamole. If you are sensitive to sulfites, you need to be a label reader and a chef interviewer. Again, keep in mind that waiters don't always know what is in the food they serve. If you know sulfites may be in some of the ingredients, avoid the food. If you suspect you have a sensitivity to food additives, report it to your physician. If you know you have a sensitivity to food additives, always carry your EpiPen and antihistamine.

Heartburn

If a food allergy doesn't get you, the acid from the food might cause a problem. Although not many teenagers experience heartburn, some do. Heartburn is the result of stomach acid backing up into your esophagus. This is sometimes called acid reflux or esophageal reflux. Not only is it uncomfortable, but it can also be an asthma trigger. One theory is that the same nerve sensors that control the reflexes in your esophagus are also active in your bronchial muscles. When the acid irritates the lining of your esophagus, it can trigger an asthmatic reaction in your lungs. Spicy foods, caffeine, high-fat foods, fruit juices high in acid, and alcohol can cause heartburn. Smoking makes matters even worse. If you have problems with heartburn, discuss them with your doctor. It may help to raise the head of your bed a few inches while you sleep. This helps keep stomach acids in the stomach where they belong. Avoid eating shortly before bedtime and try to avoid the foods that cause problems for you. Antacids and prescription medicines can help control heartburn, but be sure to discuss them with your doctor when you visit.

Aspirin Sensitivity

Aspirin sensitivity is rare in children, but it may affect as many as 2 million teenagers and adults. Those with nasal polyps and chronic sinusitis are especially at risk of having an adverse reaction to aspirin. Aspirin can cause watering eyes, sneezing, hives, an upset stomach, chest tightness, and wheezing. The reactions can be life threatening. Doctors are currently researching the cause of this reaction in people with asthma. Although no clear cause has been determined, they know that people with aspirin-induced asthma make more leukotrienes, chemicals that cause chest tightness and wheezing, than other people when taking aspirin and other aspirin-like drugs. People with aspirin sensitivity should avoid all drugs that act like aspirin including all nonsteroidal anti-inflammatory drugs (NSAIDs) such as ibuprofen and naproxen. Medicine labels may use the words acetylsalicylate, acetylsalicylic acid, salicylic acid, or salicylate instead of the word aspirin, so you must read labels carefully. Over-the-counter combination products for stomach upsets, colds, sinus pain, and general pain relief may contain aspirin. Those with aspirin senstivity may react to high doses of acetaminophen as well. If you need to take a pain reliever or something to bring down a fever, be sure to tell your doctor that you have asthma.

Teenagers, even those who do not have asthma, should not take aspirin products. Aspirin has been associated with Reye's Syndrome, a life-threatening disease that most often follows a viral infection affecting the liver and the brain. It can affect children, teenagers, and adults, but 90 percent of those affected are under fifteen. For more information about Reye's Syndrome, visit the National Reye's Syndrome Foundation's web page at www.reyessyndrome.org.

Other Drug Sensitivities

The drugs that create problems in sensitive individuals are most often used by adults. Since young people aren't taking them, they needn't worry about adverse reactions. In addition to aspirin and other NSAIDs, beta-blockers can cause asthma symptoms to get worse. These drugs are used to treat high blood pressure, heart disease, migraine headache, and glaucoma, and those with asthma probably should not take these drugs. Those with asthma need to tell their doctors they have asthma before any drugs are prescribed.

ACE inhibitors used to treat high blood pressure or heart disease have been associated with troublesome coughs that can lead to increased wheezing.

The bottom line is that some medications can be triggers for asthma symptoms. If you need over-the-counter or prescription medications, talk to your doctor about possible drug interactions.

Latex

More and more people are becoming sensitive to latex. You might not think of latex as a problem for you, but consider that it is in over 40,000 products including rubber bands and balloons! Those with allergies and asthma are more likely to develop a latex allergy.

In physicians' offices and in hospital settings, the powder inside some latex gloves helps get the latex particles into the air. Patients in hospitals and hospital workers are at the highest risk for latex allergies.

OUTDOOR TRIGGERS

Although indoor triggers can often be controlled, if your asthma is aggravated by triggers outside your home, you may not be able to control them. You can't prevent pollen from flying through the air. You can't keep mold from growing outdoors in its natural environment. You can't take the frost out of the air. Although you may be able to help reduce air pollution, you can't eliminate it. You can, however, control your exposure to it.

Pollen

People with asthma who are allergic to pollen may have increased symptoms during certain seasons. Some people are allergic to several types of pollen; others are allergic to just one. Pollens from trees, weeds, and/or grasses provoke asthma symptoms in some people. Pollens are fine, powdery, microscopic, egg-shaped, fertilization elements of

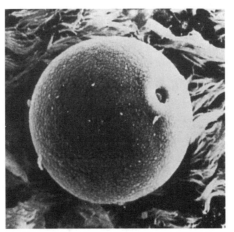

**Grass Pollen
Highly Magnified**

**Image provided by the
American Academy of
Allergy, Asthma and
Immunology**

plants. They are the male particles that must reach the female part of the plant in order for plants to reproduce. Most flowers produce large pollens that are carried by insects or birds. Unfortunately for asthmatics, tiny pollens like those in grasses and trees need the wind to help them get from place to place. These airborne pollens are the culprits that can make seasonal asthma so difficult.

Because different plants release pollens during different seasons, because the climate varies between the southern and northern regions of the United States, and because weather and temperatures aren't entirely predictable, it is hard to say when you might experience pollen-related symptoms. You might be troubled by pollen in the fall, but not in the spring, or just the other way around. Those allergic to trees are often plagued with problems in the spring (as early as January in southern states). If you are allergic to grasses, your problems could continue into the summer. If ragweed is a trigger for you, you may have problems in the late summer or early fall.

Many newspapers and television and radio stations give pollen reports during allergy seasons, and the National

Location: Philadelphia (Station No. 1), PA. Recorded: 8/26/02				
Definitions	**Trees**	**Grasses**	**Weeds**	**Molds**
LEVEL	Absent	Absent	High	Low
COUNT (m³)			76	4454
TYPE*			Ragweed	
Notes				

- Predominant allergen

Reprinted with permission from the National Allergy Bureau

The National Allergy Report presented by the American Association of Allergy, Asthma and Immunology can let you know which allergens are present in your area. This report shows that ragweed counts were high in Philadelphia on August 26, 2002. Those with ragweed allergies were probably sneezing and wheezing.

Pollen counts tell us how much of a specific allergen is in the air during a specific time. The statistics are based on the average number of allergen grains per cubic meter of air. The pollen is collected onto a sticky surface and numbers are then counted and identified under a microscope. Reports give a numerical reading (number of grains per cubic meter of air) or a count category like low, moderate, high, or very high. Pollen counts can change quickly. High winds can spread more pollen into the air and rains can wash it away. If you have specific allergies that provoke your asthma, you may want to start checking pollen counts. Remember, you need to look at the specific pollen count for your allergy. High mold levels won't affect you if you are allergic to ragweed. High ragweed allergies won't be a problem if tree pollens are high, but ragweed pollen counts are low. Many weather reports give pollen counts for the previous day, but they may also give pollen forecasts that could help you prepare. Pollen.com provides a four-day forecast for allergy sufferers. Enter your zip code and they will provide regional information.

Allergy Bureau (NAB) provides the information on the American Academy of Allergy, Asthma and Immunology's web page, www.aaaai.org/nab. (See a sample reading for Philadelphia on the previous page).

The School Asthma Allergy page will find pollen counts for your area when you enter your zip code into the "Today's Pollen Index" link, www.schoolasthma.com. Many times your local weather forecaster will give pollen and mold counts.

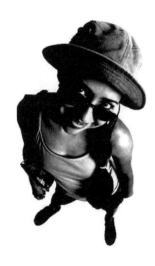

You might think you can escape your pollen-related asthma by moving to another part of the country, but unfortunately, that probably won't help. Many pollens are found throughout the United States and often those who are sensitive to one type of pollen will develop another sensitivity when they move. You can, however, escape pollens for brief periods of time by taking vacations to areas with different pollen seasons.

You can also limit your exposure to pollens by keeping windows closed when pollen counts are high and especially when it is windy. That goes for car windows, too. Limit early morning activities. Most pollens are released in the early morning. You may have to stay indoors when pollen counts are particularly high or when it is windy. Run an air conditioner if possible. It can help remove pollens from the air. Don't use window fans. A fan pulling air from outside will bring more pollen indoors and make your symptoms worse.

If you are sensitive to grass, it is probably best that you not mow the lawn or hang out outdoors while someone else in your family mows the lawn. If you do play or work outdoors, take a shower, wash your hair, and change clothes when you come inside.

If you find your asthma symptoms get worse during particular times of the year, talk to your doctor. You may be allergic to pollen. And, if despite your best efforts to follow your treatment plan and to avoid outdoor pollens, your asthma symptoms continue, you may want to discuss immunotherapy or allergy shots. Read more about this in chapter 5. Be sure to carry your fast-acting inhaler with you if one has been prescribed by your doctor.

Outdoor Molds and Yeasts

Like pollens, outdoor fungi, including molds and yeasts, are seasonal. Molds are even more affected by weather conditions, making it more difficult to predict their overall prevalence in the air. Some molds are dry and are released during dry, windy weather. Others are released in damp weather. According to the Global Initiatives for Asthma (GINA) report, alternaria and cladosporium are risk factors for asthma. Unlike indoor molds, it is impossible to clean up the mold in its natural environment.

As with pollen, it is the reproductive nature of mold that creates problems for asthmatics. The seeds or reproductive particles of molds are called spores. When the spores necessary for reproduction are released, they become airborne, and you inhale them. If you are allergic to mold and have asthma, your symptoms may be worse when mold counts are high and especially when it is windy. Outdoor molds appear in the spring and can create problems through the first frost. Just like indoor molds, outdoor molds like damp, warm places. A pile of leaves, a compost pile, a pile of rotting wood are all places where molds thrive. On farms, they often attach to grains like wheat, oats, barley, and corn, so grain bins, silos, and other storage areas are also places where molds thrive.

If you are sensitive to mold, you can take the same precautions to keep the spores from entering the house as you would with pollen. Air conditioners and dehumidifiers can help reduce humidity in your home and help prevent molds from growing indoors. Stay away from rotting materials, compost piles, etc. Carry your fast-acting inhaler if prescribed by your doctor.

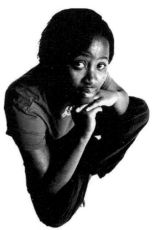

Air Pollution

Molds and pollens are airborne allergens that can provoke symptoms for many people with asthma, and air pollution may play a role as an asthma trigger as well. According to the American Lung Association, more than 142 million Americans are breathing unhealthy amounts of ozone air pollution (smog). Ozone comes from the action of sunlight on nitrogen oxides emitted in fuel combustion. The State of the Air 2002 report indicates that more than 70 percent of children who had an asthma attack in 2001 lived in areas where air quality was so poor that their counties received an "F" in air quality standards. The ten "most ozone polluted areas" are Los Angeles, Riverside, and Orange County, California; Bakersfield, California; Fresno, California; Visalia, Tulare, and Porterville, California; Houston, Galveston, and Brazoria, Texas; Atlanta, Georgia; Merced, California; Knoxville, Tennessee; Charlotte, North Carolina; Castonia, North Carolina; Rock Hill, South Carolina; and Sacramento-Yolo, California.

Ozone levels typically rise between May and October when temperatures are higher and sunlight more prevalent. People with asthma are among those at risk of breathing problems associated with smog.

Diesel exhaust may also worsen asthma symptoms. It may be the fumes themselves that cause problems or it might be that diesel particles absorb other airborne allergens and help carry these allergens into the lungs.

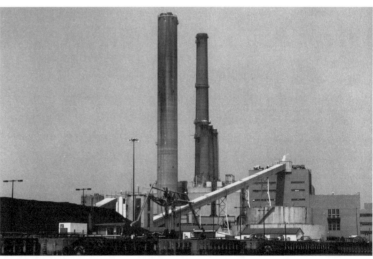

Power Plant

Photo: Penny Paquette

The Harvard School of Public Health estimates that as many as 43,000 asthma attacks in the New England area may be linked to two coal-burning power plants in the area.

TRAGIC ENVIRONMENTAL TRIGGERS

Changes in the environment can come suddenly and unexpectedly. The tragedy of the terrorist attack in New York City continues in the compromised health of those who lived and worked in the area at the time of the attack. Thousands of rescue workers from around the country continue to suffer from shortness of breath on exertion and other respiratory problems following exposure to the dust and fumes at Ground Zero. In New York City alone, up to 25 percent of the firefighters and emergency personnel are suffering from some form of illness related to exposure at the site. Some will not be able to work at the jobs they love as new exposures to smoke will exacerbate their symptoms.

Many who live in the area, those who were not directly involved in the dust cloud that followed the collapse of the buildings, also reported respiratory problems. Dr. Steven Levin, director of the Mount Sinai Medical Center, treated many people who worked in offices near the collapse. People had a variety of problems including bronchitis and lung and sinus inflammation. But according to Dr. Levine, "One of the most worrisome diagnoses is a type of environmentally induced asthma. While most upper-respiratory problems go away, this strain of asthma can stay with a person for a lifetime. . . ."

Of particular concern are the children in the area. Children breathe in more air and inhale more dust per pound than adults and their lungs are more sensitive. Three months after the attack, doctors in the area reported a surge in new and worsened asthma cases. One of the efforts of the Children's Miracle Network included donating thousands of inhalers to the Children's Aid Society. Currently, no health study for children in the area has been recommended.

FOREST FIRES

The summer of the fires, 2002, presented particular problems for those with asthma. People with asthma in the western United States had increased problems with asthma. The high levels of smoke in the air irritated their lungs and increased their symptoms. The smoke was not confined to the areas of the fires, however. The smoke spread across the country. Smoke from fires in Quebec polluted the air as far south as North Carolina, and people living in New Mexico, Nebraska, and North and South Dakota breathed smog caused by fires in Colorado and Arizona.

Doctors there advised patients to keep windows closed at night, to use air conditioner and a dehumidifier to clean the air, to keep car windows closed when traveling, to avoid outdoor exercise, to wear a paper mask when outside, and to continue to take prescribed medicines.

If you live near a power plant, you may be affected by poor air quality. A recent study by the Harvard School of Public Health reported that as many as 32 million people in New England could be exposed to pollution caused by two power plants in that area. Their study estimated that as many as 43,000 asthma attacks could be linked to two coal-burning power plants, one in Massachusetts and one in New Hampshire. While officials at the power plants say they are committed to reducing emissions at the facilities, if you live near a coal-burning power plant, you may want to join an environmental group committed to lobbying for cleaner power plants.

Weather and atmospheric conditions can create periods of intense air pollution. News and weather reports give indications of times when air quality is particularly poor. During those times, avoid unnecessary activity outside. Reduce your exposure the other inhaled allergens discussed in this chapter especially during times of increased air pollution. Again, air conditioning and air filters may help eliminate some of the problematic air particles. As in times of high pollen counts, it may be wise for your parents to time your vacation so that you will be away from your area during times of high smog concentrations. Be sure to carry your fast-acting inhaler with you if prescribed by your doctor.

Respiratory Infections

One of the most common triggers for asthma is a respiratory infection. Colds, viruses, the flu, and sinus infections can provoke asthma symptoms. Although a particular virus called respiratory syncytial viruses (RSV) cause breathing problems for infants and very young children, and may be a factor in the later development of asthma, common cold viruses are the principal triggers of wheezing in older children, teenagers, and adults with asthma. Ask your doctor for a treatment plan to follow when you get a respiratory infection and ask if you should have a flu shot.

Emotions

Have you every laughed so hard you had an asthma attack? Has a sad movie left you both sobbing and wheezing? Does your asthma seem worse when you are stressed? Doctors have been examining the role of emotions in asthma for centuries. Even Hippocrates suggested that those with asthma should avoid strong

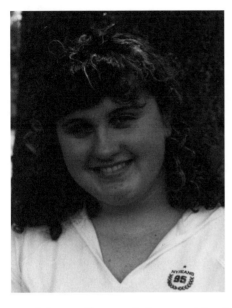

Ashley

Photo: Penny Paquette

Ashley is sixteen. She is an excellent student and likes to play field hockey, work out at the YMCA, and coach softball.

"I was just diagnosed with asthma this year. I was running during practice and got short of breath. It was very sudden. I had never had that happen before. My coach has asthma and she recognized the symptoms. I went to the doctor, and they said I was having a severe asthma attack. I was surprised. They gave me a nebulizer treatment and sent me home with new medicines, and I use those regularly now.

I find if I get a cold, it triggers the asthma. If I get a bad cold, it makes it worse. Sometimes I have to increase my medication. Besides exercise and colds nothing else seems to trigger it."

emotions. Although physicians once believed asthma symptoms were the result of emotional disorders, today they recognize that asthma is an inflammatory condition that can be triggered by many conditions. Emotional excitement may trigger asthma, but emotions don't cause it. When we laugh, cry, or yell, our breathing patterns change just as they do when we run. It may be this change in breathing that causes asthma symptoms to flare up. Changes in breathing can also happen during panic situations. It is easy to understand that someone having an asthma attack may feel anxious. At times of anxiety, rapid breathing, or hyperventilation, can occur, and that can increase asthma symptoms.

Although emotional upset doesn't cause asthma, asthma can create emotional upsets. When asthma is poorly controlled and you are unable to participate in normal activities, you may feel angry, sad, or depressed. When asthma symptoms flare up, you may feel anxious. When your parents worry about your asthma and about financial burdens that may be associated with treating asthma, you may feel upset. To learn about how other young people cope with the emotions associated with asthma, read chapter 8.

Hormones and Asthma

Hormones may also play a role in asthma attacks. Recent studies at the Medical College of Pennsylvania show that women with asthma are most likely to have severe attacks immediately before or during their menstrual periods. If you find your asthma symptoms regularly worsen just before or while you have your period, tell your doctor. This information may help in the development of your treatment plan.

Pregnancy can also change asthma symptoms. Each year close to 1 million teenage girls become pregnant. Since one in ten pregnancies is complicated by asthma, it is important to discuss your asthma with your health care specialist if you become pregnant. Changes in asthma symptoms happen in two-thirds of those who become pregnant. Your symptoms may get better while you are pregnant, but it is just as likely they will get worse. For those with milder forms of asthma, symptoms generally remain stable. Those with more moderate to severe asthma, however, may experience increased symptoms. Because poorly controlled asthma can lead to complications for mother and baby, it is essential that you monitor your asthma closely during pregnancy. The likelihood of complications is increased for smokers especially African American teens. If you are pregnant, you should consider consulting an asthma specialist in addition to an obstetrician. The specialist can review your asthma history, help monitor your symptoms, and review your medications. You may need to make changes in your medication plan during your pregnancy. Talk to your doctor about which asthma medications are approved for pregnant women.

Exercise

According to GINA, physical activity is an important trigger of asthma, and for some, it is the only trigger. For most, it is a signal that asthma is inadequately controlled. Although it is probably not wise to exercise during times of heavy pollen or mold counts, during times of significant air pollution, or during extremely cold weather, most people with asthma can and should exercise. The best method of dealing with exercise-induced-asthma is to work with your doctor to get your asthma under control.

Asthma triggers make asthma symptoms worse, but they don't cause asthma. If you have asthma, your airways are inflamed and need to be treated. You can avoid asthma triggers, and your doctor can help develop a treatment plan to keep your symptoms under control. Read more about treatment in the next chapter.

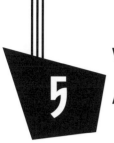

What to Do about It: Asthma Treatments

5

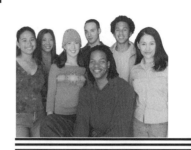

PEAK FLOW METER

The best gauge for measuring asthma symptoms is the peak flow meter. Think of it as a thermometer for measuring the severity of asthma symptoms. This device measures airflow or peak expiratory flow rate (PEFR) in what the American Lung Association calls a "fast blast." It can tell you how quickly you can "blast" air from your lungs. It can be an excellent resource in developing and following your asthma action plan. If you have more than occasional asthma symptoms, a peak flow meter can be an excellent resource.

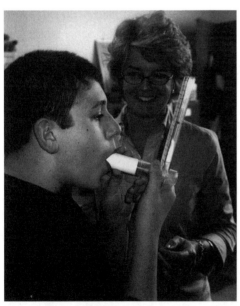

Derek using a peak flow meter

**Photo:
Penny Paquette**

The school nurse helps Derek use a peak flow meter. He says his asthma can get "really bad." He uses a peak flow meter at home and sometimes at school to monitor his symptoms, and he follows an asthma action plan developed by his doctor.

"If I am in yellow, I am cautious. If I am in red, I go to the doctor's for a treatment. The doctor wants to see what is going on if I am in the red zone," he says. Derek is thirteen years old. He likes to play basketball, ride his bicycle, and play with his dog.

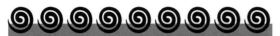

BASIC PEAK FLOW METER TECHNIQUE

▶ Slide the marker to the bottom of the scale—to zero
▶ Stand up straight
▶ Take a deep breath (the deepest you can) and place your lips around the mouth piece (don't put your tongue inside the hole)
▶ Blow as hard and as fast as you can
▶ Jot down the reading
▶ Repeat the process two more times
▶ Record the highest reading on your peak flow chart
▶ Measure your peak flows at the same time each day

Use the information in conjunction with your asthma action plan

One of the best things about the meter is that it lets you *see* your asthma symptoms. Often it can indicate increases in symptoms even before you can feel them. When you chart your readings you can get early indications of trouble and address them immediately. This can help reduce visits to the doctor's office and to the emergency room. There are different types of meters, but they all help measure your lung function. Peak flow meters cost about $20 and are sometimes available at no cost at your doctor's office.

How to Use a Peak Flow Meter

Directions for using a peak flow meter are found in the sidebar, but be sure to try yours out in your doctor's office. Your doctor or the office staff can determine if you are using it properly. You should first use your peak flow meter when asthma symptoms are under control to help determine your normal peak flow rate. You may have to record your readings for a few weeks to come up with your "personal best" result. If your symptoms aren't under control, your doctor can help your determine a temporary normal reading based on your age, height, sex, and race. Normal readings vary from person to person. Your doctor can help you determine what is "normal" for you. Once you have your normal peak flow rate, you will use it to help measure your progress.

You and your doctor will then use your measurements to determine how well your asthma management program is working. It can help you and your doctor know when it might be time to increase or change medications. The good news is, it can also let you know when your asthma is under control and may signal a time when it might be possible to decrease some of your asthma medicine. Your doctor can recommend how often you should record your peak flows. Those with the most severe types of asthma will need to record their measurements most often.

Most doctors and most peak flow meters use a "traffic light" system to interpret the readings. The readings and recommendations below are general standards developed by the National Institutes of Health. They provide you with guidelines. You should discuss your specific zones and goals with your doctors.

Green for Go

When your asthma symptoms are under reasonably good control, your readings will fall in the *green zone* of your peak flow meter, your peak flow chart, and your asthma action plan. Your readings will be between 80 and 100 percent of your personal best.

Go on with your current treatment plan and with your normal activities. Continue taking your medicine as prescribed by your doctor. If your readings stay in this green area for an extended period of time, your doctor *may* decide to gradually reduce your medication. Notice this says your *doctor* may decide to reduce your medication. Unless medication reductions are specifically outlined in your asthma action plan, don't reduce your medications without talking to your doctor.

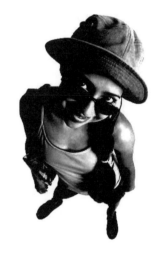

Yellow for Caution

When your readings fall between 50 to 79 percent of your personal best, you are in an asthma-warning area. Your asthma symptoms are getting worse and you need to increase your asthma medication. You should follow your treatment plan for readings in the yellow zone and step up your treatment as recommended by your doctor.

Red for Danger

When your peak flow readings fall below 50 percent of your personal best, you are in a danger area. Your asthma

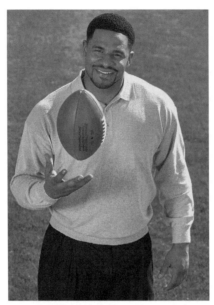

Jerome Bettis

**Photo credit:
Asthma All Star Program
GlaxoSmithKline**

2001 NFL Man of the Year Jerome Bettis has asthma. The Pittsburgh Steelers running back says he learned his lessons about asthma the hard way. He had a major asthma attack during a nationally televised game and almost died. Like many young people, he says he took his health for granted and only used an inhaler when he felt he needed to. That complacency nearly killed him.

Today he is an asthma advocate working with the Asthma All-Stars Program, a national program sponsored by five leading medical and respiratory organizations and GlaxoSmithKline. He now recognizes the importance of following a treatment plan. "I look at my asthma like the team I'm going to play against on Sunday. I train and I prepare to win. . . . The only way to get a grip on your asthma is through education, awareness, and discipline," he says.

is out of control. Your airways are narrowing and you should use quick-relief (rescue) medication immediately. If you have an asthma action plan, follow the guidelines for the red zone and call your doctor immediately.

Emergency Treatment

If your symptoms don't improve, you may need emergency medical assistance. Although you should discuss emergency treatment symptoms with your doctor, if you are in doubt, go to the emergency room. Asthma can be a deadly disease and people die each year from asthma. (Read more about this in chapter 7.) The following symptoms suggest the need for immediate medical treatment:

- ◎ **Peak flows in the red, danger zone**
- ◎ **Severe coughing, wheezing, shortness of breath, or tightness in the chest**
- ◎ **Difficulty talking**
- ◎ **Problems concentrating**
- ◎ **Shortness of breath while walking**
- ◎ **Shallow breathing—may be faster or slower than normal**
- ◎ **Hunched shoulders**
- ◎ **Nasal flaring**
- ◎ **Your rescue medicine doesn't work within 10 minutes or doesn't provide sustained relief**
- ◎ **Your lips or fingernails are blue or gray**
- ◎ **The skin around your neck, rib cage, or collar bone is sucked in as you breathe**

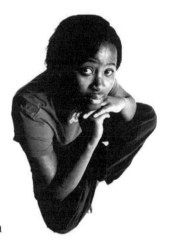

When you monitor your peak flow readings regularly, you give yourself and your doctor additional information about how well your asthma is controlled. Together you can develop an asthma action plan designed specifically for you.

ASTHMA ACTION PLANS

A personalized asthma action plan helps you and your parents manage your asthma at home. An asthma action plan is a written form developed by your doctor that gives advice formulated especially for you. It can help you determine when you should use routine medicines, and when and which medicines you should take if you have changes in your symptoms. Actions to follow are based on your symptoms and information you collect when you use your peak flow meter. Using that information, the plan outlines when and how often you should use the medicine prescribed by your doctor, when you might need to add medicine to your routine, and which medicines you should add. With a good plan developed with your physician, you will know

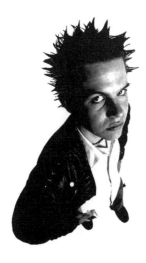

when you should call the doctor and when you should seek emergency assistance. The plan should include emergency phone numbers and the location of the hospital nearest you.

The National Jewish Medical Research Center recommends that your plan answer these five questions:

1. **When should you call your health care provider?**
2. **When should you seek emergency care?**
3. **When is quick relief medicine not enough?**
4. **If and when you should increase inhaled steroids.**
5. **If and when you should start taking oral steroids.**

A sample plan is on the next page. Many doctors use multicopy, pressure sensitive forms that provide additional copies for school personnel and others who should be aware of your condition. Your physical education teacher and your sports coaches should have copies of your plan as well. If your doctor does not provide this type of form, make photocopies for school and for close relatives. Many schools also use asthma action cards that record much of the same information. (Read more about this in chapter 6.)

An asthma diary can include the same information as well as keep track of changes in your symptoms. You can use it to record daily symptoms of coughing, wheezing, shortness of breath, chest tightness, etc. You can also use this type of plan to keep track of things that may trigger your asthma. For example, if you notice your symptoms are getting worse, you could record what you had to eat that day, what you were doing, or environmental factors that may have made you feel worse. Over time that type of record can help identify specific triggers for your asthma.

Asthma action plans and diaries can help you monitor your asthma and prevent your symptoms from getting out of control. Slight changes in your treatment can help prevent full-blown asthma episodes and can reduce the number of times you need to make visits to your doctor or to an emergency room.

SAMPLE ASTHMA ACTION PLAN

Name _____ Doctor's Name _____

Doctor's Phone _____

Nearest Hospital _____

For emergencies call 911

Asthma Triggers to Avoid _____

_____

GREEN ZONE   Peak flow readings between _____ and _____ (80–100% of best)

Good Control

      Breathing normal   No nighttime symptoms—sleeping well

      No coughing or wheezing   Use regular medicines

      Able to do normal activities

    Medicines_____Dose_____When_____

      _____   _____   _____

      _____   _____   _____

YELLOW ZONE   Peak flow reading between _____ and _____ (50–79% of best)

Caution—Symptoms Increasing

      Some symptoms during normal activities   Symptoms are increasing

      Some problems sleeping   and could cause problems

      Reliever medicine working

      Using reliever medicine up to four times a day   Step up treatment

    Medicines_____Dose_____When_____

      _____   _____   _____

      _____   _____   _____

RED ZONE   Peak flow reading _____ to _____ (<50% of best)

Danger Area

Breathing is difficult   Skin pulled in at neck, between ribs,

Wheezing even at rest   or around collarbone

Trouble moving and/or talking   Reliever doesn't help or doesn't last

Lips and/or fingernails blue or gray

SEEK MEDICAL ASSISTANCE IMMEDIATELY.

USE RELIEVER INHALER AS NEEDED UNTIL YOU GET HELP.

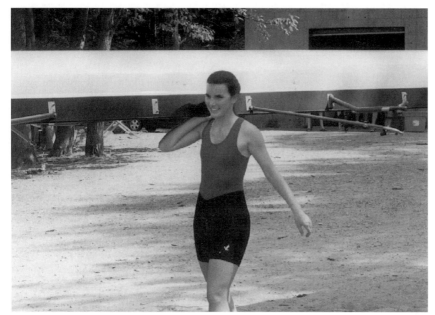

Gillian

**Photo by Mary
Ellen Smith**

Follow Your Plan

Recent studies show that teenagers don't use their inhalers as often as their doctors tell them to. Typically, young people use only 40 percent of the medicine they are supposed to use. As much as half the time, they don't use any medicine.

Elizabeth McQuaid of Brown University's Department of Child and Family Psychiatry says, "If children took medicines exactly as prescribed, asthma-related illness would decrease and quality of life . . . would increase."

Eighteen-year-old Gillian says she was among the 40 percent who don't use their medicines as prescribed. She says she didn't use her medicine as often as she was supposed to when she was younger. Unfortunately, when you don't use your medicine, you can't always do the things you want to do. Today, she says, "Take responsibility and take your medicine as your doctor prescribes."

While in high school, Gillian rowed in the eight and won the junior national pairs championship. She entered Brown University in the fall where she continues to row on Brown's crew team.

MEDICATION

The type of medicine you take and how much you take will be determined by your physician. Today, doctors recommend a "step up" and "step down" approach to manage asthma. The kind of medicine you take and how much you take will depend on the severity of your asthma. Remember, the severity of your asthma can change as symptoms increase and decrease. Your doctor will design an asthma treatment plan for you and your current symptoms.

The following provides an overview of the types of medicine that are available today. New medicines are developed each year, so this list may not include all drugs available. Each person with asthma is different with different symptoms, different sensitivities, and different responses to medicine. The information here is just that, background information. It should be use to help you have discussions with your doctor and your family about your asthma treatment.

Delivery Systems

Depending on the type of medicine prescribed by your doctor, it may be in a tablet form, a liquid inhaled through a nebulizer, in an inhaled form in a metered-dose inhaler (MDI), or in powder form inhaled through a non-aerosol inhaler. You may need to use more than one type of medicine and more than one type of delivery system. Tablets are taken the way you would any pill, by swallowing them with water. Nebulizers are machines that turn liquid medicine into a fine mist that is then inhaled through a mask or a mouthpiece. They are often used for small children and some masks are even decorated with child-friendly characters. They can also be used to treat symptoms at any age as they ensure maximal delivery of the bronchodilator medication. Most nebulizers are large and are not portable, but a new nebulizer is now on the market that can run on AA batteries or can be plugged in to a car's cigarette lighter. These newer nebulizers are small enough to be carried in a purse or a backpack.

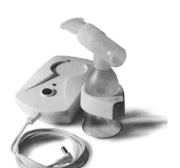

Portable Nebulizer

Photo provided by Aerogen, Inc.

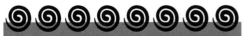

HOW TO USE A METERED-DOSE INHALER (MDI) WITH A SPACER

▶ Take the cap off your inhaler and shake well
▶ Attach the mouthpiece of the inhaler to the spacer
▶ Put your lips around the spacer mouthpiece. Press the MDI canister once to release the medicine into the spacer
▶ Inhale slowly and deeply, and hold your breath for 10 seconds
▶ Breath out slowly
▶ Repeat as prescribed by your doctor
▶ Rinse your mouth with water and spit
▶ Wash your inhaler once a week

MDIs come in a small, metal canister that is inserted into a plastic mouthpiece. Sometimes called "puffers," they deliver a predetermined amount of medicine each time you inhale. Most MDIs deliver the medicine with one or more propellant gases called chloroflurocarbons (CFCs). In an effort to help protect the environment from fluorocarbons, newer non-CFC inhalers are now becoming available. At this time, albuterol is available in a non-CFC delivery system. Other medicines will be available in this form in the near future.

According to the National Heart, Lung, and Blood Institute (NHLBI), CFC metered-dose inhalers will remain available until an adequate number of safe and effective non-CFC inhalers are available. There may be some difference in the way the new MDIs work, look, taste, or feel. According to the NHLBI, the goal is to phase out and ultimately eliminate the use of CFCs in metered-dose inhalers. If your doctor switches you from a CFC inhaler to a non-CFC inhaler, be sure to ask the doctor or the professional staff to show you the correct way to use it.

Your doctor may recommend that you use a spacer with your MDI. Spacers act as holding chambers for the medicine and help better deliver the medicine to your air chambers. Without a spacer, much of the medicine gets trapped in your mouth or at the back of your throat. A spacer allows you to take a little more time before inhaling the medicine and helps reduce some of the side effects of inhaled medicines (particularly inhaled corticosteroids. See below). Some spacers provide sound effects and make a whistling noise if you inhale your medicine too quickly. The American Lung Association reports that spacers improve the proper use of inhalers from 50 percent to almost 100 percent. MDIs are small and convenient and fit easily into a pocket or pencil case.

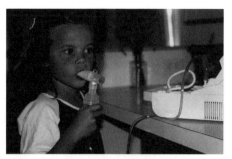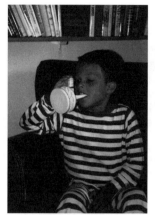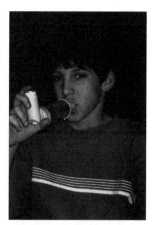

Children with age-appropriate spacers— Carlyn, Ben, and Sam with inhalers

Photos by Penny Paquette

Many young children with asthma cannot coordinate the MDI action and their breathing well enough to use an MDI. Young children often use a nebulizer instead. Nebulizers turn liquid medicine into a fine mist making it easy for young people to get the proper medicine into their airways.

As children get older, they are able to use MDIs with spacers. Younger children may use large spacers that include a whistling sound to let them know when they are inhaling their medicines correctly. By the time young people reach their preteen and teen years, most are able to use small spacers that also improve the delivery of medicines into the airways.

Some medicines are delivered in dry powder form with a dry-powder inhaler. The Turbuhaler, Diskhaler, and Diskus are trademarked delivery systems. No propellants are used in these systems. Your own inhalation delivers the medicine, and you must breath forcefully to help get the medicine into your lungs. These devices are also small and can fit into a pocket or purse. Your doctor can help you decide which medicine and which delivery system is best for you.

TREATMENT OPTIONS

Your doctor will help you decide which treatments are best for you. This is a general overview of treatment options. Some drugs may not be prescribed for children or teenagers.

Reliever Medicines

There are basically two main categories of asthma medicines. One type is designed to provide relief. It is often described as a fast-acting medication or a rescue medicine.

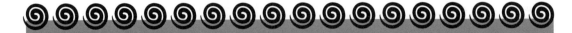

MEDICAL TREATMENTS FROM THE PAST

Inhaled medicines have been use to treat asthma since the time of Ancient Egypt when physicians burned herbs on a hot brick and asthma patients inhaled the smoke.

And remember, in the 12th century, Moses Maimonides thought chicken soup would help.

Kimberly Brubaker Bradley presents a view of 18th century asthma treatment in her young adult novel, *Weaver's Daughter*. Lizzie, a teenager with asthma, suffers some of the standard treatment of the late 18th century when the local doctor gives her medicine to purge her (make her vomit). The doctor believed this treatment would relieve her of excess phlegm.

Lizzie also gets some less drastic help from the local midwife who applies goose fat to her lips and nose and helps ease her symptoms with herbal teas. Unfortunately, these treatments do little to help Lizzie's allergies and asthma.

Myths like these about asthma treatments have been around forever. Here are a few others:

- Keep a muskrat hide, furry side down, over your chest; it will help asthma pains.
- Hold a chihuahua; your asthma will be transferred to the dog.
- For children with asthma, have the child stand against a tree. Hammer three nails above the child's head. When the child is taller than the tree, the asthma will go away.
- Bury a lock of hair below a tree stump. Once it rots, asthma will be cured.
- Catch a frog before daylight. Blow into its mouth. The frog will die before sundown and your asthma will be cured.
- Smoke a hornet's nest in a pipe and inhale the smoke
- Swallow a wad of crumpled spider's web
- Take a lock of hair, wrap it in flannel, and stuff in into a crack in the door or the floor, and your asthma will be cured.

Today modern medicines have replaced goose grease, muskrats, and chihuahuas. Your doctor can help you find a treatment that is right for you.

That's because it is intended to help stop attacks once they begin. It opens up the airways by relaxing the bronchial muscles. Sometimes it is also used to open airways before using controller medicines (see below). Your doctor may also recommend that you use it before you exercise to prevent exercise-induced asthma.

Inhaled Beta-2 Agonists

This reliever medicine is delivered through an MDI, Diskus, Diskhaler, or a nebulizer, and is called a bronchodilator because it dilates your bronchial tubes, making it easier to breath. It stimulates what is called the *beta-adrenergic receptors* on the smooth muscle of the airways and causes them to relax.

Because these medicines are inhaled, they deliver the medicine directly into the airways in the lungs. These medications temporarily relieve symptoms, but they do not treat the underlying inflammation.

Short-acting beta-2 agonists relax the airways making it easier to breathe. They act quickly, usually within minutes. They can also make the airways less twitchy and less likely to respond to triggers. They have few side effects. They can be used to relieve symptoms, to prevent symptoms before exposure to a trigger, or before using an inhaled controller medicine. Their effects usually last from four to six hours. Proventil, Ventolin, Alupent, and Brethaire are some of the brand names of this short-acting beta-2 agonist medication.

Long-acting bronchodilators are also available. They are used along with inhaled anti-inflammatory medicines and are used regularly, usually twice a day. They do not provide the immediate relief of a fast-acting bronchodilator. Their effects are longer lasting than the short-acting medicines, lasting up to 12 hours. Servent is a commonly prescribed medicine in this category. This type of bronchodilator should not be used alone. It is intended to be used along with an inhaled anti-inflammatory medicine.

Ipratropium Bromide

This inhaled medicine also opens airways. It blocks the signals from the nervous system that cause the airways to narrow. It takes up to two hours to act and cannot be used as a quick-relief or rescue medicine. It is taken on a regular basis and lasts from three to six hours. Atrovent is an ipratropium bromide medication.

These inhalers are all small and can fit easily into a pocket or purse.

All asthma medicines should be used according to your doctor's advice. Your doctor will prescribe a certain number of inhalations or *puffs* and the number of times each day you should use the medicine. Some beta-2 agonists are prescribed on an "as needed" basis for mild asthma. You use the inhaler when you need it. They are most effective when taken as soon as symptoms begin. When you begin to cough, wheeze, feel chest tighten, or feel short of breath, your fast-acting inhalers can reverse the symptoms in short order. They can also be used as rescue medicines for those with more serious asthma. Because they are so convenient and so effective, some patients overuse them. If you need to use your inhaler more often than your doctor recommends, you need to be reevaluated. You should call your doctor or an emergency room if you are having an asthma attack and your bronchodilator is not relieving your symptoms.

Theophylline

Theophylline is an oral bronchodilator, not an inhaled medicine. It, too, causes the smooth muscles of the airways to relax. This medicine is systemic. Because you swallow it and it enters your bloodstream, its effects are not limited to the airways. This medicine can cause stomach upsets, headaches, nervousness, rapid heart beat, and difficulty concentating. If you use theophylline, you should avoid caffeine as it can make side effects worse. It also interacts with some other medicines, so you must tell your doctor if you are taking any other medicines. Some theophylline medicines are quite long lasting, up to 24 hours. Take this medicine only as your doctor prescribes as overdoses can have serious consequences.

Over-the-Counter Bronchodilators

Some asthma medications are sold over-the-counter (OTC) and don't require a prescription. Bronchodilator

HOW DO YOU KNOW WHEN YOU NEED A REFILL

To be sure how much medicine you have in your MDI, you need to do a little math. How many doses are in the container? How many are you using each day? Do the math, and you will know how long your inhaler will last. Say your canister holds 200 puffs and you use eight each day. Divide eight into 200 and you will get the number of days your inhaler should last. In this example, 25 days. You can mark the date on your calendar when you should call for a refill.

If you are using a MDI for quick relief only, this system won't work. Instead, find a place to make a check mark each time you use it. A small check or dot on your calendar will work. When you near the total number of doses in the canister, call for a refill.

tablets and inhalers are both available at your local drug store and can provide short-term relief for mild asthma symptoms. The FDA says that these drugs may be effective "stopgap" measures when you don't have your prescription medicine with you, but doctors warn that OTC inhalers keep many people from getting the professional asthma treatment they need. The specific drug in these OTC products can cause irregularities in your heart rate. These medications will only treat symptoms short term and will not affect the underlying inflammatory issues of asthma.

Controller Medicines

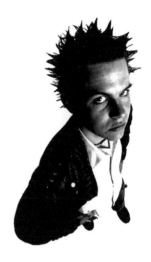

It may be that you need to add other forms of medicine to your plan daily or for a period of time. For some, a fast-acting inhaler is the only medication they need. But since asthma is a condition caused by airway inflammation, you may need to use anti-inflammatory drugs to control your symptoms.

Anti-inflammatory medications get to the root of asthma problems. Remember that upside down tree used to illustrate your bronchial tubes? Anti-inflammatories help treat and prevent the inflammation where it starts, at those roots. These are called *controller* medicines. The goal of this type of treatment is to control asthma symptoms. They are not used during an asthma attack, but are used long-term to prevent attacks from starting. They won't make you feel better right away, but over the course of treatment they will work to prevent inflammation and excess mucus.

The NHLBI recommends anti-inflammatory treatment for young people with mild intermittent, moderate, and severe asthma. In its most recent update on the treatment of asthma, the NHLBI stressed that inhaled corticosteroids are preferred for controlling and preventing asthma symptoms, and for improving lung function and qualify of life. Inhaled steroids treat chronic inflammation of the airways, which has been confirmed as a key characteristic of asthma. In the NHLBI release, Dr. William Busse, chairman of the National Asthma Education and Prevention Program, said that using the inhaled steroids in combination with long-acting beta-2 agonists "is more effective than simply increasing the dose of inhaled steroids for patients over five who have moderate or severe persistent asthma."

If you have more than occasional problems with asthma, you should discuss anti-inflammatory medicines with your doctor. There are many anti-inflammatory drugs available today. Let your doctor help you decide which is right for you.

Inhaled Anti-Inflammatory Medications

Different types of anti-inflammatory medicine may be delivered with an MDI, a Turbuhaler, Diskhaler or Diskus, or nebulizer. Often people are confused about which inhaler does what. This can be dangerous. Remember, fast-acting reliever inhalers will stop an asthma attack. Inhaled anti-inflammatory drugs do not. If you are using more than one inhaled medicine, be sure you and your family members know which is which. They may look alike, but they don't do the same things. Inhaled anti-inflammatory drugs will help keep your airways open, reduce the swelling, and decrease mucus production, but it won't open your airways quickly. Your doctor will tell you how many "puffs" and how many times each day you should use the inhaled anti-inflammatory. Some anti-inflammatory medicines are taken in pill form.

Corticosteroids

Corticosteroids have been used in the successful treatment of asthma and allergies since 1948. According to the Guidelines for the Diagnosis and Management of Asthma (GINA) report produced by the NHLBI, corticosteroids are the most effective anti-inflammatory medications for the treatment of asthma, and inhaled corticosteroids are the preferred treatment for patients with persistent asthma at all levels of severity. They improve lung function, decrease airway hyperresponsiveness, reduce symptoms, reduce the frequency and severity of exacerbations, and improve the quality of life. AeroBid, Azmacort, Vanceril, Flovent, Beclovent, and Pulmicort are among the brand names for this medication. Inhaled corticosteroids don't work immediately. It may take several days and up to a week for you to feel the benefits of the medication, so don't give up too soon. As with all medications, use your inhaled steroid as your doctor prescribes and follow your doctor's recommended management plan before increasing or decreasing the medication. Inhaled corticosteroids are often used after a quick-relief medicine. The quick-relief medicine opens the airways to allow the inhaled corticosteroid to better enter the airways. Most doctors recommend using a spacer with inhaled corticosteroids. Because the drug can cause a sore throat and sometimes thrush (a yeast infection in the mouth), you should always rinse your mouth after using this medicine.

Unfortunately, corticosteroids are sometimes confused with the anabolic steroids inappropriately and illegally used by body builders and other athletes. Corticosteroids are natural substances that can fight respiratory inflammation. Anabolic steroids are related to the male sex hormone, testosterone. Although they are legally prescribed for some health conditions, they are not the drugs used in asthma prevention.

Another cause for concern with inhaled corticosteroids has been its effect on growth in young people. Fortunately, this concern was addressed at the 58th Annual Meeting of the American Academy of Allergy, Asthma and Immunology (AAAAI) in March 2002. Doctors presented the results of recent research indicating that while growth may be slowed during the first year of inhaled corticosteroids treatment, it does not have any long-term effect on growth. Although the doctors suggested that the growth of young people taking these drugs should be monitored, long-term data indicate there is no effect on final height. Even at low doses, inhaled corticosteroids help many young people sleep better, improve the ablility to exercise, decrease the use of fast-relief medication, and help patients avoid visits to the emergency room. There may be very slight differences in growth rates for different inhaled corticosteroid drugs. You can discuss which might be best for you with your doctor.

> Recent studies suggest inhaled corticosteroids have no long-term effect on growth in young people.

Recent research at Boston's Brigham and Women's Hospital show an increased risk of bone loss among premenopausal women who are using inhaled steroids. The amount of bone loss increased as the doses (or number of puffs a day) increased. Although the yearly losses were small, there may be some increased risk of hip fracture in those who use inhaled steroids long-term. While you are young to be thinking about this, you may want to keep it in mind as your asthma treatment continues.

Research in the area of bone loss continues. What doctors do know for sure is that inhaled steroids are of significant benefit in treating asthma. While the bone loss relationship continues to be studied, researchers who did the study recommend using the lowest dose of inhaled steroids necessary to control symptoms. According to the National Institutes of Health report, those who combine inhaled steroid treatment with long-acting beta-2 agonists are able to reduce the number of inhalations of inhaled steroids necessary to control symptoms. Talk to your doctor about bone loss studies and about the levels of inhaled steroid use that will be best for you.

Inhaled Nasal Steroids

In addition to inhaled steroids for your bronchial tubes, doctors may recommend using inhaled nasal steroids. These are often used in patients who have sinus congestion and/or allergic rhinitis associated with asthma.

Oral Corticosteroids

Oral corticosteroids given either in a tablet or syrup form or by injection are sometimes used for short-term (three to ten day) periods. Doctors sometimes call this a steroid "burst." This type of burst helps patients regain control of asthma symptoms during serious episodes. Prednisone is one of the most commonly prescribed steroid drugs for asthma patients. Methylprednisolone and Prednisolone are also oral corticosteroids. Like the inhaled medication, these drugs decrease the swelling in the bronchial tubes and help reduce mucus. Used for brief periods of time, they have no major side effects. Since asthma can be fatal if uncontrolled, the condition itself is a much greater risk than a short course of steroid treatment.

Sometimes, however, it is necessary to take oral steroids for longer periods of time. Doctors usually only recommend long-term use of steroids when all other treatments fail. If your doctor recommends the long-term use of oral steroids, be sure to discuss the possible side effects which can include weight gain, cataracts, decreased growth, high blood pressure, elevated blood sugars, and the thinning of bones and skin. Still, if you need them to breathe, you will need to take them. Your doctor will monitor you for possible side effects.

Cromolyn and Nedocromil

Cromolyn (Intal) and nedocromil (Tilade) are also prescribed as anti-inflammatory controller medicines. They keep the airways from swelling and prevent mucus production when you are exposed to an asthma trigger. Like inhaled steroids, they cannot reverse an asthma attack once it has started and are used to prevent symptoms from developing. In order to prevent symptoms, your doctor may recommend you use them everyday. Sometimes, they are also prescribed as a pretreatment before exercise or before exposure to a specific asthma trigger. Then, the medicine is used five to fifty minutes before exercise or exposure. The effects of the treatment last for several hours. Cromolyn is available in MDIs, in powder form, and as a liquid for nebulizer treatment. Nedocromil comes in an MDI.

These medications must be taken regularly to be effective. They do not act immediately and the benefits increase gradually over weeks and months of use.

Sometimes patients experience a dry cough after using these medications. You should rinse your mouth after treatment.

Leukotriene Modifiers

Prescription drugs Accolate, Singulair, and Zyflo (zafirlukast, montelukast, zileuton) are leukotriene modifiers, the newest class of anti-inflammatory drugs. Leukotrienes are chemicals in the body that are associated with airway inflammation, constriction, and the accumulation of fluid in the lungs. These oral drugs fight asthma by interrupting the activities of these chemicals, preventing them from causing the symptoms associated with asthma. They help prevent exercise-induced asthma and asthma triggered by allergies. They also seem to reduce symptoms in those with aspirin sensitivity. When they are added to an inhaled steroid treatment they make it possible for patients to reduce the amount of inhaled steroid they need to control symptoms. They are used in the treatment of chronic asthma. This medicine is used to prevent symptoms, not to treat an asthma attack once it has started. They are taken regularly. Some of these drugs can interact with drugs used to prevent blood clots. Tell your doctor about any drugs you are taking before starting any new medication.

Combination Medications

The Advair Diskus combines a long-acting inhaled bronchodilator and an inhaled corticosteroid to treat asthma. The dry powder delivers twelve hours of protection. It is not, however, a fast-relief medicine and should not be used to treat an asthma attack. You will still need a fast-acting bronchodilator for rapid relief of symptoms. These medicines can irritate your throat and cause hoarseness. To prevent these side effects, rinse your mouth after using.

Cautions: A recent survey by the American Lung Association found that 73 percent of adults did not know the difference between controller medicines (those that prevent symptoms) and reliever medicines (those that can alleviate an attack). Even more parents of asthmatics were confused—79 percent. Make it your business to know the difference.

Immunotherapy

Immunotherapy (allergy shots) is sometimes recommended for those who have allergy-induced asthma. When the major cause of asthma is an inhaled allergen that can't be avoided, allergy shots may help. Some studies indicate that immunotherapy may also be effective in helping prevent those with allergies from developing the disease.

Allergy shots stimulate the body's immune system. When an allergen is injected into your body, the immune system handles it in two ways. Special T-cells in the immune system release chemicals that signal the immune system's B-cells to stop making an allergic antibody to the injected substance. The T-cells also stimulate the B-cells to produce an antibody that can neutralize and block the antibody before it can trigger an allergic reaction. Doctors inject patients with a weak solution of the specific allergen or allergens that cause allergy and asthma symptoms in that individual. The vaccine is developed for a specific individual and includes an extract of the specific allergen that causes problems for that individual. Gradually, the strength of the allergen is increased.

Doctors have been using immunotherapy since the early 1900s.

Immunotherapy has been used to treat allergic symptoms for nearly a century. In 1911, allergy researchers Drs. L. Noon and J. Freeman injected hay fever patients with an allergy extract of grass pollen before hay fever season began. They noted that their patients had fewer symptoms during grass pollen season. Today, immunotherapy, or allergy shots, are used to treat allergic conditions including asthma, hay fever, and sensitivity to stinging insects.

Patients have shots once or twice a week for several months until they reach the highest recommended dose. This maintenance-level dose continues, but the length of time between shots gradually increases to a month between treatments.

Patients must wait in the doctors office for about a half hour after receiving the injections to be sure they will not have an adverse reaction.

These shots gradually decrease the patients sensitivity to the substance—grass pollen, ragweed pollen, birch pollen, mountain cedar pollen, dust mites, cat dander, dog dander, and/or mold spores. According to the National Jewish Medical and Research Center, the nation's leading treatment center for respiratory diseases and immune disorders, doctors may recommend immunotherapy for those with very specific allergens who don't respond well to traditional treatment or those who have symptoms throughout the year.

The NHLBI of the National Institutes of Health says immunotherapy can be risky and potentially life threatening and should be considered only after other strict avoidance of allergens and drug interventions have failed to help.

AFFORDING TREATMENT

Many young people with asthma have difficulty following their doctor's recommendations because their families simply can't afford to buy medicine. If your family is struggling financially, you may not be getting the daily treatment you need. Those in low-income families are some of the hardest hit by asthma and are the most often hospitalized. Many drug companies now offer free prescription medicines to those who cannot afford them. According to the Allergy and Asthma Network: Mothers of Asthmatics (AANMA), the pharmaceutical industry gave away nearly $1.5 billion worth of prescription to 3.5 million patients in 2001. The Pharmaceutical Research and Manufacturers of America offer a directory of assistance programs. Visit the Web site www.phrma.org/pap for more information or call the toll-free number 1-800-762-4636 for a copy of the directory. Your doctor can help you complete the necessary paperwork to qualify for these programs.

Additional Medications

Your doctor may prescribe additional medication for sinus problems, heartburn, or allergies that will be used in conjunction with your asthma medicine to help prevent and control your symptoms.

CURRENT RESEARCH

Doctors continue to look for better ways to diagnose and treat asthma and they continue to look for ways to prevent it.

Bacteria

This year, researchers reported that a bacteria that causes pneumonia may also contribute to the development of asthma. A type of pneumonia that can stay in the lungs long after a person has appeared to recover may play a role in asthma. Researchers at the University of Texas Southwestern Medical Center in Dallas recently found that 78 percent of mice infected with the bacterium developed asthma-like qualities in their lungs eighteen months after they were infected.

Another study found that many patients with asthma may have bacterial infections in their lungs that respond to antibiotics. Researchers at the National Jewish Medical and Research Center reported that more than half of the chronic, stable asthmatics in the study showed evidence of infection with mycoplasma or chlamydia bacteria. The lung function of those with the infection improved significantly following treatment for the infection. Doctors said it isn't clear how the bacterial infection influences chronic asthma, but it might not only exacerbate the disease but contribute to the development of the disease as well. Doctors in the study cautioned against the widespread use of antibiotics to treat asthma, but said doctors might consider it for those who do not respond to even the maximum doses of standard medication.

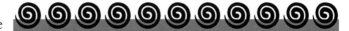

EXPERIMENTAL TREATMENTS

A new anti-IgE therapy is undergoing clinical trials at this time. Researchers have designed a drug to block immunoglobulin E (IgE) before it binds to mast cells. This interrupts the chemical reaction (histamine) responsible for allergy symptoms. Anti-IgE attaches to IgE in the blood and prevents the release of histamine and the allergic reaction.

Rather than reversing symptoms or reducing inflammation, this new therapy would prevent the allergic reactions that cause the symptoms. This could prove to be an exciting new form of treatment for those with asthma. In testing, the therapy reduced asthma episodes in patients with moderate to severe allergic asthma. It also allowed patients to reduce or eliminate use of inhaled corticosteroids. The new drug known as Rhumab-E25 is delivered by injection under the skin. In the tests, the new drug was administered every two to four weeks, depending on the patient's weight and IgE level. This drug may be approved for treatment by the time you read this book.

According to the American Academy of Allergy, Asthma and Immunology, researchers and clinicians are trying to find the genes that predispose individuals to asthma. This is a difficult task as there are no universally accepted definitions of asthma or specific indications as to why asthma occurs only in certain people. Without this information there is no way to scientifically identify inherited disorders or predict how they will respond to therapy. Genetic research may provide answers in asthma diagnosis and treatment in the near future.

Researchers in England and the United States may be on the track of an asthma gene. They have found that a defective gene, called ADAM 33, is related to the development of overresponsive airways associated with asthma. Researchers are very excited about the discovery and believe it could lead to new ways of diagnosing and treating asthma.

Allergic Rhinitis

Allergic rhinitis was recently proven to have a strong link to other respiratory diseases including chronic sinusitis, middle-ear infections, nasal polyps, and asthma. Researchers are now exploring these relationships and looking at ways to determine which patients with allergic rhinitis are at the highest risk for developing asthma. They are exploring several theories to explain the relationship between asthma and allergic rhinitis including a similar anatomy theory. The anatomy of the tissues in the nose and lungs are almost identical. Both are exposed to the same allergens and irritants and respond in similar ways. They are also looking at the nasal-bronchial reflex. This view explores the idea that there are nerve fibers originating in the upper airway that connect to the lungs. This allows an allergic reaction in the nose to cause a reflex reaction in the lungs. Nasal blockage is also being examined as a link. When nasal passages are blocked by allergic rhinitis, it is necessary to breathe through the mouth. This mouth breathing may trigger asthma symptoms. Postnasal drip of inflammatory material is probably a trigger for asthma. Researchers continue to look at the link between the inflammatory chemicals commonly found in the noses of people with allergic rhinitis and the inflammation of the airways in asthma. Some researchers believe asthma and allergic rhinitis may be the same disease.

The development of new information in treating, diagnosing, and preventing asthma continues each year. If you have found your asthma particularly resistant to treatment, don't give up hope. New treatments are just around the corner.

CURRENT NEWS

For current news about asthma, check the American Academy of Allergy, Asthma and Immunology's "What's New" section of their home page www.aaaai.org.

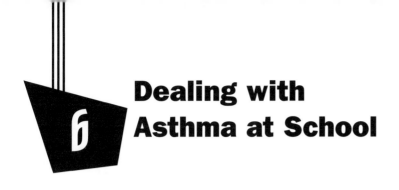

Dealing with
Asthma at School

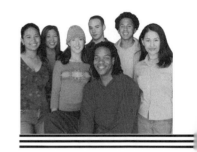

Since young people spend most of their days inside a school or traveling to and from school, the school environment can play an important role in asthma management.

NOTIFYING SCHOOL PERSONNEL

Classroom teachers, gym teachers, coaches, school nurses, and school administrators should know if you have asthma. Most schools will help organize an asthma management plan and an emergency response plan specifically for you. Many physician-provided asthma action plans are made of pressure-sensitive paper with a copy designed to go to school personnel. Some school nurses have similar forms available. The Asthma and Allergy Foundation of America provides a Student Asthma Action Card like the one on the following page on their Web site at www.aafa.org. In many school systems, students are required to have an asthma management plan on file if they want to carry a metered-dose rescue inhaler on them.

SCHOOL ENVIRONMENT

Unfortunately, school environments are sometimes hazards for young people with asthma. Dust, chalk dust, art supplies, classroom pets and their saliva and urine, laboratory and cleaning chemicals, and smells can all be triggers for asthma. Mold contamination is so severe in some buildings that they have had to close permanently. Carpeting in schools can complicate problems by providing a desirable environment for dust mites and mold.

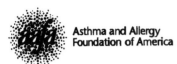 **Asthma and Allergy Foundation of America**

STUDENT ASTHMA ACTION CARD

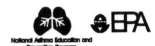
National Asthma Education and Prevention Program

Name:_____ Grade:_____ Age:_____

Homeroom Teacher:_____ Room: _____

Parent/Guardian   Name: _____ Ph: (h): _____

                         Address: _____ Ph: (w): _____

Parent/Guardian   Name: _____ Ph: (h): _____

                         Address: _____ Ph: (w): _____

ID Photo

Emergency Phone Contact #1_____
                              Name   Relationship   Phone

Emergency Phone Contact #2_____
                              Name   Relationship   Phone

Physician Treating Student for Asthma: _____ Ph: _____

Other Physician:_____ Ph: _____

EMERGENCY PLAN

Emergency action is necessary when the student has symptoms such as, _____ , _____ ,

_____ , _____ or has a peak flow reading of _____ .

• Steps to take during an asthma episode:

   1. Check peak flow.

   2. Give medications as listed below. Student should respond to treatment in 15-20 minutes.

   3. Contact parent/guardian if _____

   4. Re-check peak flow.

   5. Seek emergency medical care if the student has any of the following:

       ✔ Coughs constantly

       ✔ No improvement 15-20 minutes after initial treatment with medication and a relative cannot be reached.

       ✔ Peak flow of _____

       ✔ Hard time breathing with:
          • Chest and neck pulled in with breathing
          • Stooped body posture
          • Struggling or gasping

       ✔ Trouble walking or talking

       ✔ Stops playing and can't start activity again

       ✔ Lips or fingernails are grey or blue

IF THIS HAPPENS, GET EMERGENCY HELP NOW!

• Emergency Asthma Medications

Name	Amount	When to Use
1.		
2.		
3.		
4.		

See reverse for more instructions

DAILY ASTHMA MANAGEMENT PLAN

- **Identify the things which start an asthma episode (Check each that applies to the student.)**

☐ Exercise   ☐ Strong odors or fumes   ☐ Other _____

☐ Respiratory infections   ☐ Chalk dust / dust   _____

☐ Change in temperature   ☐ Carpets in the room

☐ Animals   ☐ Pollens

☐ Food _____   ☐ Molds

Comments _____

- **Control of School Environment**

(List any environmental control measures, pre-medications, and/or dietary restrictions that the student needs to prevent an asthma episode.) _____

_____

_____

_____

- **Peak Flow Monitoring**

Personal Best Peak Flow number: _____

Monitoring Times: _____ _____ _____ _____

- **Daily Medication Plan**

	Name	Amount	When to Use
1.			
2.			
3.			
4.			

COMMENTS / SPECIAL INSTRUCTIONS

_____

_____

FOR INHALED MEDICATIONS

☐ I have instructed _____ in the proper way to use his/her medications. It is my professional opinion that _____ should be allowed to carry and use that medication by him/herself.

☐ It is my professional opinion that _____ should not carry his/her inhaled medication by him/herself.

_____   _____

Physician Signature   Date

_____   _____

Parent/Guardian Signature   Date

AAFA • 1233 20th Street, N.W., Suite 402 , Washington, DC 20036 • www.aafa.org • 1-800-7-ASTHMA

02/00

Reprinted with permission of the Asthma and Allergy Foundation of America

101

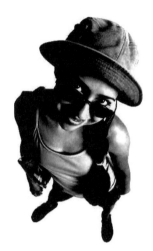

Schools should have no-smoking policies to assure a smoke-free environment for all students and school personnel.

The Environmental Protection Agency (EPA) provides kits for schools to help them manage indoor air quality. Cosponsored by the National PTA, National Education Association, Council for American Private Education, Association of School Business Officials, American Federation of Teachers, and the American Lung Association, the kit can help school personnel improve indoor air quality at your school. If your school is not already using this plan, perhaps your student government association can work with your school's parent organization to encourage your school to clean up its act with this handy kit. The kit provides schools guidelines for general cleanliness, pest control, animals in the classroom, drain traps in the classroom, moisture and mold in classrooms, temperature, ventilation, exhaust fans, art supplies, science supplies, industrial and vocational supplies, and locker rooms as well as special procedures to help identify and protect young people with asthma. Your school can get information about this kit on the EPA's Web site www.epa.gov/iaq/schools/scholkit.html.

SCHOOL ASTHMA MANAGEMENT PLANS

You should have an asthma action plan to help you treat your asthma symptoms. Your school should have its own asthma plan to help inform school personnel and to assist students in keeping asthma symptoms under control. In the treatment section of the book, we discussed multicopy reports that can help schools treat students with asthma. The school nurse should have a copy of your personal plan.

Schools should have their own management plans as well. These plans cover the school's role in helping young people with asthma. All school personnel should be given asthma information. This should include not just classroom teachers, but coaches, food service personnel, bus drivers, administrators, janitorial staff, etc. Anyone who comes in contact with students should be knowledgeable about asthma.

The school should be aware of specific triggers for students with asthma and school officials should have procedures for seeing that you can take your asthma medication at school including whether you may carry your own medication and equipment—inhalers, EpiPens, peak flow meters (see below). If you need a nebulizer treatment, are nebulizers available at your school? Who will assist with nebulizer treatments? Do you need to supply your own medication cup and/or tubing?

Your school should have an emergency plan for all medical emergencies including severe asthma episodes. School personnel should have a plan for dealing with emergencies whether they occur in the classroom, the gym, the school cafeteria, or the athletic field. School personnel should be aware of students who have serious asthma in order to help them if a serious episode happens. Ask your school nurse or school administrator if your school has a plan.

Five million young people in the United States have asthma. Schools should have nurses to help treat them while they are in school. Nurses in schools do more than dispense medicine. Nurses can help identify students with asthma, implement a student's asthma management plan, supervise medical equipment needed to treat students, and provide adult support to young people with asthma. Although the National Association of School Nurses recommends one school nurse for every 750 students, only six states meet this recommended level of staffing. In some states, the ratios are as high as one nurse to every 10,000 students. And, even in those states with ideal nurse-to-student ratios, nurses must cover more than one building. Most nurses cover 2.4 schools. On average, school nurses care for more than 1,000 students, and at least 53 students of them have asthma.

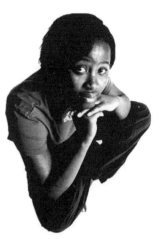

Although much of the professional literature recommends that school nurses monitor young people with asthma, in reality, school secretaries and school teachers are often assigned the task of treating students including dispensing medicine. In some schools, clerical workers and teachers have refused to be responsible for dispensing medicine. In a recent study by researchers at the University of Georgia, 78 percent of teachers surveyed said they feel unprepared to teach children with a chronic illness such as asthma. A recent *Asthma Magazine* survey of school nurses reveal that they, too, believe teachers are ill prepared to supervise asthma treatment of their students. Forty-two percent of the nurses surveyed said a lack of teacher/staff knowledge about asthma was a problem. Researchers in the study recommended that school nurses may be able to customize training for teachers to help prepare them to monitor and treat asthma.

What can you do in this situation? Be sure you are informed. Know about your asthma, what triggers your episodes, and what treatments work best for you. If your state allows you to carry your own medication (see below), have it with you at all times. Most professionals acknowledge that by the time young people reach their teen years, they are mature enough to handle their own medicine at school. Find out who is responsible in your school for assisting students with asthma. Your parents should meet with that person at the beginning of the school year to review your asthma management plan. If no school nurse is available to help implement your plan, be sure your doctor uses language that non-professionals can understand when writing up your treatment plan. If you need nebulizer treatments during the school day, find out where you will receive your treatments and who will be responsible for supervising those treatment at the start of the school year.

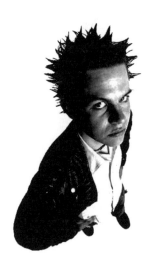

MEDICATIONS IN SCHOOL

One of the most important factors in controlling asthma symptoms may be your school's position on carrying medications in school. Concern over drugs in schools has provoked many schools to take a hard line regarding medicines in school. Recent surveys indicate that many school administrators and teachers don't recognize the severity of asthma.

Many schools require that asthma inhalers be kept in the nurses office or in the school office. The American Academy of Allergy, Asthma and Immunology (AAAAI) believes this puts young people like you at risk. Their doctors believe that preteens and teenagers who can recognize their symptoms and know how and when to use their inhalers should be allowed to carry an inhaler prescribed by their doctor. They and many medical professionals say keeping prescribed inhalers in the nurse's office can delay necessary life-saving treatment during an asthma attack. When doctors prescribe rescue inhalers, they usually come with directions for the patient to carry the inhalers with them at all times. Specialists caution that asthma attacks can happen anywhere—at lunch, at recess, during a field trip, in the classroom, in gym. According to the Allergy and Asthma Network: Mothers of Asthmatics (AANMA), when schools refuse a young person the right to use an inhaler, it puts students at risk of what could be a life-threatening asthma attack. It also puts other students at risk of watching a dangerous event. Teenagers who have been taught the proper use of an inhaler should be allowed to

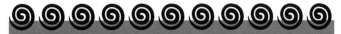

VIRTUAL CHILDREN'S HOSPITAL

Children's Hospital of Iowa's Virtual Children's Hospital (www.vh.org) has this to say about students self-medicating with inhalers:

School policy restricting possession of medication by students is insufficient grounds for preventing students with sufficient maturity from retaining possession of their bronchodilator inhaler. Such policies, when enforced, delay appropriate treatment, restrict activities unnecessarily, and require that the student be identified among peers as requiring special attention. The decision regarding sufficient maturity of the student to be responsible for appropriate inhaler use is an individual one to be made by the parents in consultation with their physician. The inhalers pose no abuse potential or other danger to classmates. It therefore constitutes unreasonable interference with the student's medical care for school personnel to unilaterally restrict possession of bronchodilator inhalers by students judged by parents and physician to have sufficient maturity to use the device appropriately. While restrictions on bronchodilator inhaler possession may be necessary for the youngest students, the earlier students begin to take responsibility for their own inhaler use, the earlier they will be able to manage their asthma sufficiently to function in a fully peer-appropriate manner and thereby minimize feelings of difference from classmates. This feeling of control and self-confidence is important in the long-term management of asthma. Possession of the bronchodilator inhaler by the student also promotes earlier use that decreases the risk of requiring emergency medical care from rapidly progressive asthma, which on rare occasion can cause hypoxia, brain damage, and death.

Miles Weinberger, M.D.
Professor of Pediatrics
Director, Pediatric Allergy and Pulmonary Division
www.vh.org/Patients/IHB/Peds/Allergy/Asthma/
13School.html

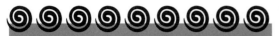

According to the Allergy & Asthma Network/Mothers of Asthmatics, the following states have policies allowing students to carry and use inhalers in school:

Delaware—1999
Florida—2001
Georgia—2002
Illinois—2001
Kentucky—2002
Louisiana—1994
Massachusetts—1994
Michigan—2002
Minnesota—2001
Missouri—1996
New Hampshire—2003
New Jersey—2001
New York—2001
Ohio—2000
Oregon—1997
Rhode Island—1998
Texas—2001
Virginia—2000
Wisconsin—1999

Legislation in each state varies, and many schools have specific requirements for students and their parents before allowing students to carry inhalers. Check with your school board for the requirements in your school system.

carry it with them. Often, students with exercise-induced asthma need to use an inhaler before an athletic practice or competition. Too often teens find it embarrassing and inconvenient to have to visit the nurse's office or the school office before gym class, practice, or competitions, and they choose to try to exercise without using their prescribed inhaler. This puts them at increased risk.

Most often when young people treat an asthma attack immediately, symptoms can be reversed. Although asthma deaths in young people are rare, people have passed out at athletic competitions, died getting on buses, and died at athletic events when inhalers weren't readily available. It might seem sensible to keep inhalers in the nurse's office, but nurses aren't always in their offices. In many school systems, one school nurse covers several schools and are often on the move from one to another. Unfortunately, many schools do not have onsite nurses at all. In some schools, clerical help is sometimes expected to keep track of asthma medications.

Representatives of the AANMA spoke on Capitol Hill recently to advocate changes in school policies regarding inhaler use. AANMA President Nancy Sander said, "Our kids are mandated to attend school, yet for students with asthma, school can be a very dangerous place. Every year, children die of asthma at school and on field trips."

When the goal of asthma management plans is to help young people recognize if and when they need to use their inhalers, it makes sense to allow properly trained teens to treat their own symptoms.

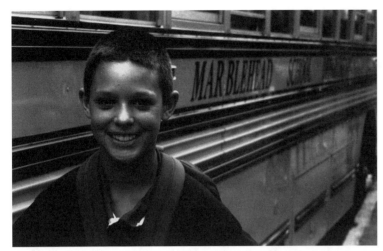

Alex

Photo: Penny Paquette

Students like Alex are placed at risk when school buses idle while waiting for students. Diesel exhaust can irritate airways and provoke asthma attacks.

Thirteen-year-old Alex was diagnosed with asthma when he was five. He is allergic to pollen and dust and says his asthma is sometimes worse when it is very hot and humid. He likes to play with his dog, play video games, and just hang out. He also likes to play soccer, though he is sometimes bothered by his asthma when he plays.

The states listed in the sidebar on the previous page allow students to carry inhalers in school. The most recent state added to the list is New Hampshire where on January 31, 2003, lawmakers passed legislation to allow children with asthma or allergies to carry their own inhalers or epinephrine at school and camp. Check with your school to see what requirements you must meet in order to carry your asthma medicine in school or check the AANMA site at www.aanma.org/cityhall/ch_childrights.htm and click on your state to find your local requirements. If your state is not on the list, discuss it with your parents and together work to advocate for a change in your state's policies.

SCHOOL BUSES

If you ride to and from school on the bus, you may face an additional asthma trigger. According to a recent Yale University study, students who ride buses inhale exhaust fumes about 180 hours each year. Diesel exhaust can irritate your airways and cause asthma attacks.

The problem seems to be at its worse during pick up and drop off times. With engines idling, the fumes can cause problems for students waiting to get onto the bus or waiting for friends after they have gotten off the bus.

GYM CLASS

Many students with asthma have problems in gym class. Sometimes physical education teachers confuse asthma symptoms with those of an out-of-shape student. They see the breathlessness as a signal that the student needs more physical exercise to get in shape, when in fact the breathlessness is caused by airway restrictions. Sometimes even students with asthma think they are out of shape when they can't complete certain exercise tasks.

Many students mention that running the mile, which is part of the Presidential Physical Fitness Test, is a struggle that they must face each year at least once in gym class. Some are humiliated when despite their best efforts they can't complete the mile, or even worse, push themselves into an asthma attack in order to meet the challenge. A student who could run a mile in the middle of the summer might have seasonal asthma problems in the fall or in the spring. Students who have outdoor allergies can often complete this challenge with less of a problem if they run indoors.

The National Heart, Lung, and Blood Institute of the National Institutes of Health suggests that students may sometimes need to have their programs modified by varying the type, length, and/or frequency of activity. This doesn't make you a wimp and it doesn't mean you aren't fit. It simply recognizes that when your asthma symptoms aren't under control, you just can't get enough air to complete the activity.

When asthma is under control, most students should be able to participate in physical education activities. However, those with exercise-induced asthma may need to use an inhaler before exercising. Physical activities that are sustained, like long periods of running, are more likely to provoke asthma symptoms. Still, many athletes with asthma complete activities that require intense exercise. With well-managed asthma, you should be able to take part in all activities.

ATTENDANCE POLICIES

Ten million school days are lost each year because of asthma. These include sick days as well as days missed for diagnosis, treatment, and evaluation of asthma. Poorly managed asthma keeps young people home more often than necessary.

If you have serious asthma that keeps you out of school, you should have a plan to help you keep up with school work. Don't wait until you have missed school to deal with the issue. Plan ahead. Work with your parents and teachers to develop a strategy to help deal with missed school days and assignments.

When students aren't allowed to treat themselves for their asthma symptoms, they lose even more time. If you need to use an inhaler only once each day, but you need to go to the school nurse to do it, the AANMA says you lose an additional eleven days over the course of the school year.

Some schools have strict attendance policies that can penalize young people with chronic medical conditions like asthma. Sometimes schools allow waivers for students who must miss school because of illness or for treatment.

Many teenagers with asthma have nighttime symptoms that keep them from sleeping well at night. Although asthma conditions may seem improved in the morning, fatigue from the previous night's struggle to breathe can affect attendance and performance. Researchers at Johns Hopkins University found that the more times young people wake up at night, the more likely they are to miss school.

Many students miss a lot of school during the early stages of evaluation and development of treatment plans. Until your doctors find a treatment plan that keeps your symptoms under control, you may be one of those students contributing to the 10 million school days lost.

Ten million school days are lost each year.

Once an individual asthma action plan is in place, school attendance should improve. If you need help deciding whether or not you should go to school, the AANMA provides the following guidelines:

If you have a runny nose, mild wheezing that clears after treatment, can do normal activities, and don't have trouble breathing, you should go to school. If you have an infection (sore throat, swollen glands), a fever over 100 degrees, wheezing that doesn't respond to treatment, weakness or fatigue that makes it difficult to do normal activities, or you have trouble breathing, you should stay home. Use your peak flow meter to help measure your breathing ability and follow your asthma treatment plan to help evaluate your symptoms.

If you have severe asthma and must miss a lot of school, your school may provide a tutor. Contact your school's special education department to find out if you qualify.

If you have a medical condition that keeps you out of school, ask if your school has attendance waivers.

FIELD TRIPS

When you travel away from school, you can't be certain what triggers you may be exposed to. Take your inhaler and/or EpiPen with you. If your school does not allow you to carry your own medicines, be sure someone on the trip will carry them for you.

Students with asthma should be able to go on most school-sponsored trips. If your asthma is under control, most school trips should not present problems. You know your triggers and you know what trips might present problems. A trip to a saw mill might present problems if you are sensitive to sawdust and wood products, for example. A trip to a horse farm may present problems if you have an animal allergy. If you carry your prescribed quick-relief medicine with you, most trips should not be a problem.

Day trips are not the only concern for teens, however. By the time students are in high school, many take trips far afield. Foreign language trips to Europe, student exchanges to other countries, cultural trips to other lands are not uncommon. If you are going to be traveling out of the country, you need to meet with your doctor to discuss what precautions you need to take while on your trip. Your doctor can prescribe both routine and emergency medicines to take with you. This may include antibiotics and steroids in addition to your usual medicines. Be sure to take your medicine in your personal carry-on bag or backpack. Don't put medicine in checked baggage that could be delayed or lost. Carry your medicine in the original container that lists directions for taking it. Take your peak flow meter and a current asthma action plan that includes the details of your condition, a list of your current medications (include generic names), and when you should take them as well as your normal peak flow readings. If possible, bring back-up medicines or at least written prescriptions for replacements and have someone else carry them in case yours are lost.

If you need to use a nebulizer, there are portable models available that run on batteries. Otherwise, you will need electrical adapters. Find out what you will need to make your nebulizer work in the countries you will be visiting.

If you are in the middle of immunotherapy, getting your shots on schedule may be difficult. You will need to arrange for a professional to administer your shot and to supervise you for a least 20 minutes after the injection. You will also need to bring injectable epinephrine with you in case of an adverse reaction to the allergy shots. Allergy extracts need to be refrigerated at all times and they need to be labeled with your name exactly as it appears on your passport.

Your parents will need to write a letter designating an adult on the trip to act on your behalf in case of an emergency. The letter should be notarized.

Be sure your traveling companions, chaperones, and any family you stay with know you have asthma and how to deal with it in an emergency.

There is more cigarette smoking in many foreign countries than in the United States and it may be more difficult for you to avoid this trigger. If you will be housed with another family, be sure to request a non-smoking family.

Domestic flights are all non-smoking, but some international flights are not. If you will be flying out of the country, be sure to request seating in a non-smoking section.

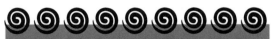

PHYSICIAN REFERRALS

The American Academy of Allergy, Asthma and Immunology's (AAAAI) Physician Referral and Information line, 1-800-822-2762, can provide the name of an allergist that practices in the area you will be visiting. You can also visit the physician referral system online at www.aaaai.org.

SELF-ADVOCACY

As you enter your high school and post-high school years, you will need to take more responsibility for your asthma management. This will include advocating for yourself if you have particular needs. When you visit your doctor, review your asthma action plan. Be sure you can describe what asthma is, what triggers your asthma, what can be done to avoid triggers, and what treatments you need to manage your symptoms. Once you have that information, you will be in a better position to work with teachers and coaches at your school to ensure you get the necessary treatment or accommodations to keep you safe.

When Asthma Becomes Deadly

7

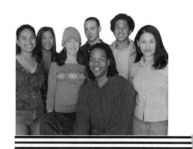

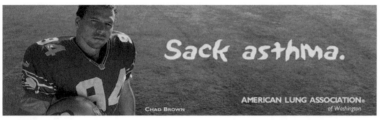

Chad Brown

Poster provided by the American Lung Association of Washington

Chad Brown of the Seattle Seahawks learned he had asthma after collapsing during a football game in 1988. He says the diagnosis came as a surprise, but also a relief. He had been trying to ignore the asthma symptoms and was worried because he hadn't been able to compete with his usual intensity. It turned out the allergens in Seattle were different from those in Pittsburgh where he had played previously.

Today, Chad Brown serves as a spokesperson for the American Lung Association of Washington. He says his medications now open up his lungs and allow him play. He was named to the AFC Pro Bowl Team two years in a row.

Many people don't recognize the seriousness of asthma and find it hard to believe that people actually die from it. Most don't believe an active young person could have a fatal attack. Unfortunately, that's just not true. Although asthma deaths are rare in young people, they do happen. In 1998, 5,438 people died from asthma. Another 6,850 people have asthma listed as a contributing cause of death on their death certificates. Two hundred and forty six children under age 17 died from asthma that year. On average, 14 Americans die each day. Although the death rate is the highest among African Americans—more than double that of white Americans—and more females die of asthma than males, people of all backgrounds can die from a serious asthma

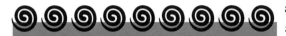

RECENT ASTHMA DEATHS AMONG YOUNG PEOPLE

▶ An 18-year-old collapsed in a school hallway after playing softball in a physical education class. He died at a local hospital less than two hours later. (2002)

▶ A 10-year-old died waiting to board the school bus. (2001)

▶ A 33-year-old actress died in her apartment following a catastrophic asthma attack. (2001)

▶ A 34-year-old boxing champion died of complications from asthma. (2002)

▶ A 13-year-old girl died from an asthma attack and one of her kidneys was donated to her father. (2002)

▶ A 16-year-old who loved baseball and playing the guitar died of brain damage and cardiac arrest following an asthma attack. (2001)

▶ A 14-year-old boy died following an asthma attack at summer camp. His inhaler was locked in the infirmary because laws in the state prohibit campers from carrying prescription medicines. (2002)

attack. Certain risk factors make asthma-related deaths more likely (see chart), but it is important to know that it can happen to anyone.

Most asthma deaths follow a gradual increase in asthma severity, often following a respiratory infection, and could probably have been prevented if adequate treatment procedures were followed. Some severe episodes, however, come on suddenly and death can result within minutes. Doctors call this sudden asphyxic asthma. If treated quickly, even those with this type of asthma can survive.

EMERGENCY PROCEDURES

Unfortunately, asthma can get out of control. Sometimes people with asthma don't have access to proper medical care or can't afford the daily asthma medications that could help. (For information about drug companies that provide medicine at reduced rates or for free, see chapter 5.) Those without health insurance often wait until asthma symptoms are so serious that they require an emergency room visit before seeking treatment. Some people ignore their doctor's advice and don't take their medications as prescribed. Teenagers often fall into this category. Whether it is because they don't want to believe they have asthma, they don't want to use inhalers in front of friends, or they don't like the way the asthma medicine makes them feel, young people are at high risk of what doctors call noncompliance, or not following the doctor's advice. This is particularly risky. The death rates among all asthmatics nearly doubled between 1980 and 1993. For teenagers, the death rate quadrupled!

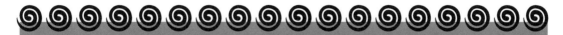

PATIENTS AT HIGHEST RISK OF ASTHMA-RELATED DEATH

Age

- Late teens
- Early 20s
- Over 55

Ethnicity

- All ethnicities at risk, but greater risk for African Americans

Severe Asthma History and Hospitalizations

- History of sudden, severe asthma
- Hospital admission within the past year
- Multiple emergency care visits
- Prior intubation for asthma
- Prior admission to intensive care
- Prior near-fatal attacks
- History of seizures

Family Problems

- Poor family support
- Family problems including alcohol abuse, depression, family loss, unemployment, etc.
- Patient in denial

Complicating Health Problems

- Serious psychiatric illness
- Extreme anxiety
- Illicit drug use
- Cardiovascular diseases
- Other chronic respiratory diseases
- Life-threatening allergies

Beta-2 Agonist and Oral Steroid Use

- Use of more than two canisters per month of rescue inhaler
- Current use of oral steroids or recent withdraw from oral steroids

Problems Accessing Immediate Medical Care

Other Factors

- Poor understanding of disease, its effect on airflow obstruction, and its severity
- Sensitivity to alternaria (an outdoor mold)
- Low socioeconomic status and urban residence

Especially For Teens

- Denial
- Failure to recognize asthma symptoms
- Forgetfulness
- Belief that medicine is ineffective, inconvenient, or cumbersome
- Fear of side effects of medicines
- Peer disapproval
- Reluctance to get medical treatment

Note: It is important to know that anyone can die of a serious asthma attack. This chart shows the risk factors that are often associated with death.

Sometimes even those who follow their asthma management plans have serious asthma episodes that require emergency-room care.

If you have an asthma action plan, you will have guidelines to help you decide when a visit to the hospital is in order. This information is generally in the red section of most asthma management forms. It will indicate exactly what you should do in case of an emergency, including what medicine to take and how much to take. It will outline when you should call the doctor and when you should seek emergency assistance. If you don't already have an asthma action plan, talk about developing one with your parents and your doctor.

Everyone who has asthma knows what it feels like to have an asthma attack. Most often, asthma symptoms are quickly reversed with a fast-acting bronchodilator or rescue inhaler.

Sometimes, however, rescue inhalers don't relieve symptoms and breathing difficulty gets worse. Most often, asthma symptoms worsen gradually over the course of a few days, but sometimes serious episodes come without warning. If you have asthma, it is best to have a plan for emergencies

Some people with asthma also have allergies that can cause anaphylactic reactions. Certain foods, drugs, insect stings, latex (sometimes found on exercise equipment), and sometimes strenuous exercise combined with another factor can cause a severe reaction. If you have this type of allergy, you should carry an EpiPen (a prepackaged adrenaline injection). You should also have one in your home. Make sure everyone in your family as well as close friends and relatives who visit often know where the EpiPen is. If you are exposed to an anaphylactic trigger, follow your doctor's instructions for an emergency. You will probably use the EpiPen and maybe an antihistamine and call 911 for help.

Just as schools should have a plan for treating asthma emergencies, you should have one at home. During an asthma emergency, your doctor may want you to take

EMERGENCY SIGNS IN ASTHMA

- ▶ Severe coughing, wheezing, shortness of breath and/or tightness in the chest
- ▶ Difficulty talking or concentrating
- ▶ Walking causes shortness of breath
- ▶ Breathing is shallow and fast or slower than usual
- ▶ Shoulders are hunched
- ▶ Nostrils expand with breathing
- ▶ The neck area and the area between or below the ribs move inward while breathing
- ▶ The skin turns gray or blue, beginning around the mouth or under the fingernails
- ▶ Peak flow numbers fall in the danger zone
- ▶ Rescue medicine does not provide relief or only provides relief for a short period

EMERGENCY SIGNS IN ANAPHYLAXIS

- ▶ Tingling sensation or itching
- ▶ Hives
- ▶ Swelling of throat and mouth
- ▶ Difficulty breathing
- ▶ Abdominal cramps, nausea, vomiting
- ▶ Weakness
- ▶ Disorientation
- ▶ Collapse and unconsciousness

If *any* of these symptoms occur, seek emergency medical treatment right away. Follow your doctor's advise for using your bronchodilator or EpiPen.

repeated puffs of your rescue inhaler until you get help. If you have a spacer, use it. It makes the medicine easier to inhale and delivers more of it into your airways. Your doctor may recommend taking oral corticosteroids if you have them on hand. If you don't respond to your medicines, your doctor will probably want you to come to the office or go to the emergency room.

Talk to your parents about what you and they will do if you have a serious asthma attack and what you will do if you are not with them. Make a plan ahead of time.

In 1998, asthma was the cause of 2 million emergency room visits—867,000 were young people under 17. Your doctor may advise that your parents drive you to the hospital, but there are times when emergency treatment means calling an ambulance. Emergency technicians are experienced in dealing with asthma and can help care for you even before you get to the hospital.

> In 1998, 867,000 young people received emergency room treatment.

Create a form with your doctor's name and phone number, a list of your regular allergy medicines, the location of the nearest hospital, the phone number of a friend or relative who can watch your siblings if your parents need to take you to the hospital or you need to go in an ambulance, a list of the medicines and dosages you usually take. This will help your parents in an emergency and anyone who might be at your house to help you if you parents are not at home.

IN THE HOSPITAL

Hundreds of thousands of teenagers visit hospital emergency rooms every year. If you go to the hospital, here is what will probably happen there.

They will take a quick history including a review of the symptoms listed in the emergency treatment box. (If you are unable to talk, your parents can take care of this.) They will want to know what medicines you usually take and what special medicines or doses you used before coming into the hospital. (This is where the list comes in handy.)

Chapter 7

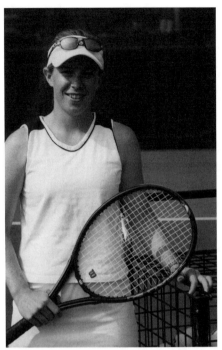

Katie

Photo: Penny Paquette

Katie was about to enter her sophomore year in high school. She was enjoying her summer and looking forward to playing in soccer competitions during her break from school. Her asthma was acting up though. Her chest felt tight and she knew from experience that she would probably need a breathing treatment and some prednisone if she wanted to compete on the weekend. Her doctor was out of the office, so she opted to go to the emergency room. She had been there before for treatment. Having had asthma since she was two, she was familiar with the emergency room. She always responded very well to the breathing treatments she got there and usually felt better within four hours of having a steroid medication.

What happened to Katie once she got to the hospital was something she could not have imagined.

"I went to the emergency room and got a breathing treatment and it didn't clear things up. I felt tight. Usually I had steroids right away, but I had been exposed to chicken-pox a few days before and they were reluctant to give me steroids. After my second breathing treatment, I got tight and that made me nervous because I usually respond well."

Unfortunately, Katie didn't respond well this time. Her airways continued to tighten and doctors needed to sedate her, put a tube down her throat, and connect it to a respirator to help her to breathe. Katie says she remembers going into the trauma room and vomiting. She doesn't remember what happened after that. But she now knows what happened.

"They airlifted me by helicopter to another hospital because I wasn't getting any better. When I got to the hospital, I went into pulmonary arrest. Fortunately, they got my heart and lungs working again, but then my blood pressure dropped. It was bad."

Katie didn't wake up until the next day. She remembers that she could not talk because of the respirator and her arm was very swollen from the medications she had received through her IV. She saw her father who was holding a clipboard so she could write down what she wanted to say.

"Then I just drifted in and out of sleep. The experience was like running a marathon sitting down. My heart rate went up to 180 at one point. The doctors were amazed I got through it. I was very fortunate."

Katie recovered from the episode, but she was a long way from recovered. She spent a year on oral steroids and needed to use a nebulizer three times a day. She wasn't allowed to participate in any physical exercise for a month and then was only allowed to go for walks. That was very hard for her because she played soccer, tennis, and basketball while she was in high school. Eventually though, she was able to return to her athletic activities. She says she monitored her peak flows very carefully, took her nebulizer treatments between classes, and was especially cautious when she got a cold. Even the sniffles could trigger an asthma episode. One of the hardest things for her was having to take steroids.

"Taking prednisone for a long time was difficult. It plays with your emotions, your appetite, and your weight. Still, it is a miracle drug when you need it."

She had a couple of minor episodes during her junior year, but has not required breathing treatments, steroids, or hospitalizations since her senior year.

"I've learned a lot. When I was younger, I had a lot of trouble managing my asthma. I didn't like to tell my mom when I was not feeling well. I didn't want her to limit my activities. Then, things would get worse. Slowly I have learned that isn't the best way to treat this. I can go down very quickly. Fortunately, I can respond quickly if I take care of it right away. I know I have to be very careful when I get a cold. Even a head cold can make my asthma worse. I am aware of that and I monitor my peak flow very closely."

Katie now has her asthma under control. She just graduated from college and will be the soccer coach at a New England college in the fall. She is spending her summer teaching tennis.

Depending on the severity of your symptoms, they may do a peak flow test and/or blood tests (see sidebar) before they begin treatment, or they may do them during treatment.

They will probably give you oxygen to help you breathe and they will have you use an MDI with a spacer or a nebulizer to help inhale a fast-acting beta-2 agonist or rescue medicine. They may have you use the MDI or nebulizer several times within an hour. Depending on the severity of your symptoms and your response to the treatment, they may also give you oral corticosteroids to help reduce airway inflammation. They will repeat breathing tests to monitor your improvement. Most people respond to this emergency treatment and are released from the hospital after a few hours with a plan to help reduce the likelihood of additional emergency visits.

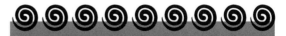

IF I AM HAVING TROUBLE BREATHING, WHY DO I NEED A BLOOD TEST?

When red blood cells pass through your lungs, 95 to 100 percent of them become "saturated" with oxygen. During an asthma episode, fewer cells become saturated and less oxygen is delivered to your organs. Doctors can measure your level of distress and your level of improvement by monitoring your oxygen saturation levels. Often this is done with an instrument that clips painlessly to your finger called pulse oximeter. It provides an estimate of your oxygen saturation.

Another test sometimes used to measure oxygen saturation is an arterial blood gas measurement. A technician will draw a blood sample from an artery, usually the one in your wrist. The blood is then tested for its oxygen level.

Sometimes, however, initial treatment does not significantly improve the asthma episode. In that case, you may be admitted to the hospital where professionals can treat your symptoms more aggressively. In addition to continuing nebulizer or MDI treatments, you may need to have stronger medicines injected directly into your veins. This is called IV or intravenous injection. This treatment delivers the medicine directly into your bloodstream. If you still do not improve, it may be necessary to have a machine help you breathe. The doctor will place a flexible plastic tube into the trachea to ventilate the lungs. The tube will be connected to a ventilator, a mechanical device designed to help patients breathe. Under these conditions, you may be looked after in the intensive care unit of the hospital until your symptoms improve. As your breathing improves, your doctor will gradually reduce the mechanical airflow until you are able to breathe on your own. Once your breathing is stabilized for a few days, you will probably be able to go home.

Emergency treatment for asthma is a clear indication that your treatment plan is not working. The emergency staff will send you home with a short-term treatment plan, but you must call your doctor for a reevaluation. It will be important to know what made your asthma worse. Were you taking your medicine as directed? Did you follow the course of treatment for increased symptoms? Were you exposed to something you are allergic to? Your doctor will review your asthma history and will develop a new treatment plan to help you get your asthma under control and keep it under control. This would be a good time to review your inhaler and peak flow meter techniques as well.

PREVENTION

Use your asthma action plan to attack your asthma symptoms when they get worse. You may need to step up your medicine until your symptoms are controlled again. Once asthma gets out of control, it is harder to reduce symptoms. The best way to avoid an asthma emergency is to prevent one.

Coping
with Asthma

8

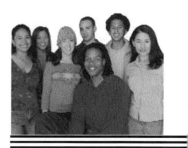

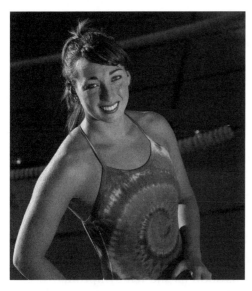

Amy Van Dyken

Photograph courtesy of the Asthma All-Star
Program and GlaxoSmithKline

Champion swimmer Amy Van Dyken has had asthma since she was a little child. She says she started swimming in hopes of relieving some of her asthma symptoms. "I was one of those kids who couldn't go out to recess and play. I couldn't go on field trips. If I ran, I couldn't breathe."

Amy calls herself a "severe asthmatic." She says she grew up hearing about all the things she couldn't do. She couldn't go out and play; she couldn't be around dust; she couldn't run. Even success at swimming came slowly. She started swimming when she was six years old, but couldn't swim the length of the pool until she was twelve.

She says learning to cope with her asthma has given her enormous drive and that she now knows that "the things you can't do are much less important that the things you can do. . . ." She says without that drive she probably would have stopped competing after winning four gold metals in the 1996 Olympic Games. Instead, she competed again in 2000 on the world record-breaking 400 meter relay team.

Amy has some advice for those who are struggling with asthma. She says, "my advice is not to let anyone hold you back and to follow your own dreams, and to always aim for the stars . . . because if you fall short you will land on the moon and there aren't too many people on the moon!"

Medical treatments can help prevent and treat asthma symptoms, but what about your feelings? How does having asthma make you feel and how can you deal with those emotions.

People with asthma respond differently to the diagnosis and to living with the condition. Depending on the severity of the problem, the length of time they have had the illness, the response to treatment, and how much they know about asthma, responses vary. Think about how you feel. Young people I talked to described denial, confusion, depression, frustration, guilt and shame, anger, feelings of being different, helplessness, fear and on a positive note, relief.

DENIAL

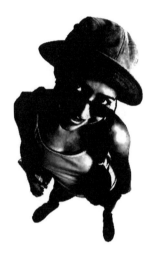

Some people who are diagnosed with asthma, including many teenagers, deny the problem. They reason that if they don't have a problem, they don't need to take medicine. Many young people find it hard to believe that anything bad could ever happen to them. They are young, healthy, and strong. They don't want to take medicine everyday. Some say they find it cumbersome and inconvenient. Some don't want to use inhalers in front of other people.

A young woman from England told me that she didn't always use her inhaler as soon as she felt symptoms coming on especially if she was with friends. "I waited until I could find a private place to do it, such as a restroom, or I would wait until I get home. My friends didn't laugh at me or anything. I just didn't like doing it." She said she has learned from an unfortunate experience, however. "I used to ignore my symptoms, but once my Mum found me collapsed in the bedroom and I had to go to hospital and be intubated. I would rather not repeat that experience, so I do everything, well almost everything, my doctor tells me to do."

Another young person said, "I would not accept that there was anything wrong with me and ignored the advice to take any inhalers. I felt fine. It was only when I ended up in the hospital that I began to accept that I might have a problem. . . . Looking back, I had been coughing every night for weeks," he said.

As these two young people learned and as you read in the previous chapter, denial can be a dangerous thing. So many very successful people have learned to live with their asthma and the treatment necessary to keep their symptoms under control. Look at the list of people in chapter 2. Anyone can have asthma. The difference in how you feel depends greatly on how well you treat it. Just as some people accept that their vision isn't terrific and they need to wear glasses or contact lenses if they want to see and enjoy life, those who accept their asthma and treat it as their doctors recommend find their lives are improved. With proper treatment, they can do all of the things they enjoy. As one young man I spoke to said, "If people think it is weird that I have to use my inhaler, that's their problem, not mine."

CONFUSION

Some people with asthma make an attempt to treat their condition, but confusion gets in the way. Many inhalers, both reliever and controller types, have similar shapes. Depending on the brand they could be gray, white, orange, or blue. As you read in the treatment section, if you use a controller inhaler during an attack, you will not get any relief. If your doctor has prescribed both a reliever and a controller inhaler be sure you know which one is which. Sometimes generic inhalers are a different color than their name brand prescription counterpart. If you get an inhaler and it looks different, check with your pharmacist to be sure you have received the correct medicine, and then to help you remember which is which, put a mark on the quick relief inhaler. This will help you keep them straight. Carry a rescue inhaler with you.

You can keep your controller medicine with your toothbrush. Since many controller inhalers are used once or twice a day, putting the inhaler with your toothbrush will remind you to use it, and you will be near a sink and can rinse your mouth after taking your puffs. Some newer combination medicines come in a different shaped delivery system that is helping with some of the inhaler confusion. If you use a reliever medicine before using your controller medicine, ask your doctor for an extra reliever inhaler so you can keep one with your toothbrush and one in your purse, pocket, or backpack.

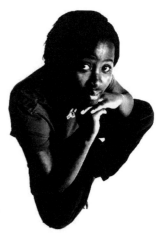

EMOTIONS AND ASTHMA

In the late 1800s, many doctors believed that asthma was a psychological disorder caused by emotional upsets. Today doctors know that asthma is a medical condition caused by airway inflammation. Emotions don't cause the disorder, but emotional ups and downs can provoke an asthma episode.

Because we breathe deeply and quickly when we laugh or cry, these changes in breathing patterns can sometimes trigger asthma episodes just as breathing changes with exercise can provoke an asthma attack. So, the changes in breathing cause the attack, not the emotions.

Researchers in Baltimore believe that emotions can also predispose the body to asthma exacerbations. Doctors there studied twenty-four children while they watched *E.T. the Extra-Terrestrial*. They monitored the children's heart rates and oxygen saturation levels and found changes in them during the sad portions of the film. The doctors believe the study shows that children who are sad or depressed may be more vulnerable to asthma attacks.

Sometimes people panic during an asthma attack. The fear and anxiety resulting from the attack causes them to breathe more quickly or hyperventilate. That further stimulates the airways and makes the attack worse. Although asthma attacks can be frightening, it helps to try to stay calm.

If you are confused about your medicines, be sure your doctor or the office nurse reviews all your medications with you before you leave the office. Information can rid you of confusion.

I FEEL DIFFERENT

Maybe you feel different from your peers. Perhaps you think having asthma makes you stand out from others your age. Often young people who have had to miss a lot of school because of asthma feel this way. They feel isolated from classmates and sometimes find themselves falling behind in school. This just makes matters worse. The good news is current asthma treatment is able to keep most young people in school. Having a plan for make-up work before asthma episodes strike has helped others. Some people find support groups helpful.

One young man mentioned that he couldn't visit his friends' homes as most of them had pets. He thought that was a bit of nuisance, but said his friends were willing to play outside or come to his house to hang out.

As with many things, the best defense is a strong offense. If you are worried about how having asthma will affect your social life, take the offensive. Tell people you have asthma. Explain to them that with the proper treatment it doesn't have to affect your activities. They, however, may need to make some adjustments in their lives. If they are truly your friends, they will make adjustments without hassling you.

Smoking is a biggie. Most teenagers don't smoke, but many do. Tell your friends that cigarette and marijuana smoke make your asthma worse. If you don't feel

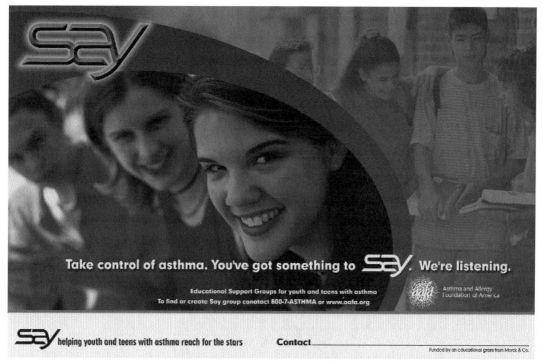

Poster reprinted with the permission of the Asthma and Allergy Foundation of America.

Support for Teenagers

The Asthma and Allergy Foundation of America sponsors support groups for adolescents called *SAY Groups* where young people have a chance to talk to other people their age about the challenges they face every day. You can find more information about this program and a group near you on the AAFA Web site www.aafa.org or call 800-7-ASTHMA for more information.

The American Lung Association recently launched a chat room for teens with asthma. You can share your feelings and concerns with others at the Lung Lounge Chat Room. You can register with the American Lung Association Web site at www.lungusa.org/press/asthma/lounge.html.

comfortable encouraging them to quit, at least let them do you the favor of quitting when you are around.

Perfumes and aftershaves can present problems in social situations, too. If you meet someone new who you plan to spend more time with, tell him or her that you have asthma and that certain scents can trigger your symptoms. Be straightforward. Tell them you know how to manage your asthma and that it is not a big deal. Explain the steps you take to prevent and control your symptoms, and that some smells, while pleasant for most, are actually a trigger for you. It is better to let a new friend know in advance than to

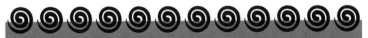

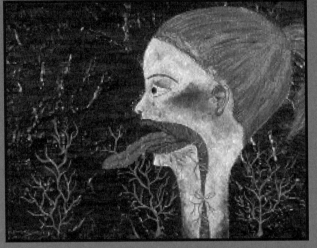

This artwork by Julieanne was one of the winning entries in the Youth Section of "Living with Asthma" art competition, a joint initiative of Asthma Australia and AstraZeneca Australia. All winning entries can be viewed at www.asthmaaustralia.org.au.

Breathe, breathe nice and slow, don't you think I'm trying,
In and out, out and in, it's hard to breathe
Under water, everyone knows that, yet,
Everyone still looks, they all come and look
Leave me, unless you can help me, so just
Leave me, listen, try and listen to my pain,
The waters rising, and I'm going down
Deeper, deeper into the ocean, why won't
Someone save me? I don't like the sea, the further
Down you sink, the less life there is. Not
The mask, I hate the mask, all scuba
Divers have to wear a mask, but mine is
Always put on late, when I'm already in the
Water, what if one day, it comes too
Late? I'll see the ocean floor, the dead
Dark, ocean floor.
Lifeless
I don't want that
I just want to breathe
Is that a big request?
I just want to *live* . . .

find yourself sitting in a car filled with perfume or aftershave gasping for air. Think about it, which is really more embarrassing?

Going out? Take your reliever inhaler. Unexpected activities, odors, or environments could trigger an attack. Be prepared.

Going dancing? Dancing is exercise and exercise can trigger asthma. If you use a pre-exercise asthma medicine, take it with you and use it before you hit the dance floor.

AFRAID AND OUT OF CONTROL

Many people who have just experienced their first asthma attack are fearful. Let's face it, not being able to breathe is a pretty scary experience. One middle-school student told me, "An asthma attack feels kind of scary—pain in the chest—have to slow down and get some air. It feels freaky. I was afraid the first time."

Julieanne a young Australian woman wrote about her fear. Read her poem on this page.

For those who have to go to the hospital for the first time, especially those who have needed to go by ambulance, the experience leaves them shaky and worried. Education and experience helps most through this fear. As you learn more about your asthma, what triggers it, and how to control it, you begin to feel that you are more in control of the situation. If, however, you are still feeling fearful, talk to your doctor about it. Some find it helpful to join a support group. One young woman shared her experience attending a support group. "It was really hard to start with, talking to people I had never met before, but when we began talking, all the things they felt about their asthma were the same as mine. It really helped me come to terms with my problems. I've made some new friends as well!"

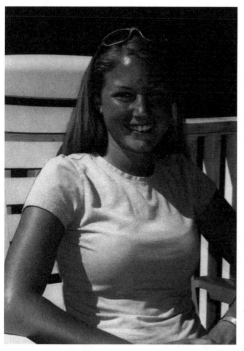

Michele

Photo: Penny Paquette

Michele, a recent college graduate, now works as a teacher for young people with special needs. She has had serious asthma most of her life. She says she got very upset when she couldn't do the things she wanted to do.

"I hated having to stop things. I loved soccer. I feel asthma is a lot of the reason I was not better. I loved it and could have done more with it if not for asthma. I played wing, but I had to come out every five minutes."

Michele still needs to be on medications all of the time. Often, she needs to use a nebulizer and takes it with her when she travels. Although it takes fifteen minutes away from things she would rather be doing, she says it is worth it. "If I don't use it, I can't do the things I want to do. . . . You can't let it beat you," she says.

Another young woman said she felt better once she started using her peak flow meter to monitor her breathing. She said the readings gave her a better understanding of how she was doing and made her feel more in control of the situation.

ANGER

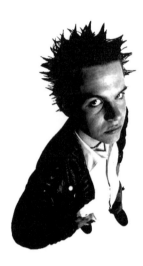

Many young people feel angry about having asthma. Most of the angry teens are upset because asthma sometimes gets in the way of the things they like to do—riding bikes, playing soccer, running the mile, skiing. For most, the anger is a short-term response to a relapse. Most people with asthma have occasional flare-ups that get in the way of activities they enjoy.

It is reasonable to be upset when you can't do the things you want to do. If your anger about asthma extends beyond the times when your activities are restricted, talk to someone. Talk to your parents, your friends, or a nurse or counselor at school. Sometimes just talking about it with someone can help make you feel better. Maybe you are not a talker. Some researchers have found that those who write about their emotions feel better. Try keeping a journal.

DEPRESSION

Occasionally, the anger, guilt, frustration, sadness, and fear are just more than some people with asthma can deal with. They may feel sad, angry, or frightened most of the time, not just during asthma episodes. Sometimes asthma comes on top of other problems in their lives. Family problems, girlfriend or boyfriend problems, or problems with school work added to a health problem makes it difficult to handle emotionally. If you are feeling overwhelmed by these feelings for extended periods of time, it is important to get help. Talk to your parents. Meet with your doctor. Talk to a counselor at school. These people can listen to you and guide you to other professionals who specialize in helping young people get through these difficult periods.

MY PARENTS WON'T LEAVE ME ALONE

A common complaint among teens is that they want to be left alone. They can manage their asthma, they say. They don't need nagging parents to remind them. As you get older, you should expect to begin taking over your medical decisions. You will be leaving home soon and it is important that you understand what causes asthma and how to treat it. Your parents, however, want to be sure you are healthy and safe. They know that life-threatening episodes are rare, but that they do happen. They want to protect you. How can you find the balance between wanting to take over your asthma and keeping your parents "off my back," as one young person put it?

One way to take control of your asthma is to follow your treatment plan. At your next doctor's visit, you do the talking. Ask your parents, in a nice way mind you, to let you talk to the doctor. Let them know you are grateful to have them be an extra set of ears for you, but that you want to have a conversation with the doctor. Ask your questions—the ones that have been troubling you. Whether it is a concern about using a steroid medicine, whether there is another medication that might be more convenient for you, or how to best handle preexercise treatment, whatever it is, you ask the questions. Allow time for your parents to ask questions when you are finished.

Some young people have found it useful to make contracts with their parents. Most often, these involve using a peak flow meter and keeping a record of readings. If you can show your parents that your readings are in the optimal range for your asthma (the green zone), that will help them relax a little. By the same token, if you let them know when your readings are falling and how you plan to treat your symptoms as a result, they will be impressed with your level of responsibility.

GUILT AND SHAME

Although asthma is no one's fault, sometimes people feel guilty about having it. Even though it isn't rational to feel guilty about having asthma, it doesn't stop people from feeling that had they done something different, they wouldn't have asthma. Often parents feel guilty about a child's asthma. Sometimes young people with asthma feel guilty because they take so much of their parents' time. Doctor's visits, even routine visits, take time out of their parents' days, they reason. Sometimes they worry about finances. Without insurance, asthma is an expensive condition.

"I don't like being sick. . . . It is embarrassing having to use an inhaler. . . . I don't like feeling like an invalid," are typical responses to having asthma. "I have seen people turn around to use their inhalers. They don't like people watching," one 13-year-old told me.

These are just some of the things young people say about having asthma. They actually feel ashamed of having

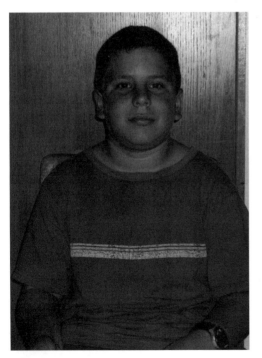

Michael

Photo: Penny Paquette

Eleven-year-old Michael says asthma can get "boring." "I cough, I wheeze, sometimes I am short of breath. I mind wheezing the most because it keeps me up at night."

He says he tries not to use his inhaler in front of people. "People react and that makes me mad and annoyed," he says.

He finds it especially annoying when people react to his coughing. "I am used to coughing, it is normal for me, but my teacher has asthma too, so when I cough she says, 'Why don't you get a drink of water?' or 'Are you okay to go to the nurse?' She worries too much."

Michael likes to play soccer. He says he can't play forward because that requires too much running, but he likes to play in goal because he likes the action. He also enjoys taking trips with the Boy Scouts.

the illness as if somehow they are at fault. When it comes time to run the mile, they are ashamed that they can't do it. When they have to step out of a game to use an inhaler or catch their breath, they are ashamed. They begin to feel that they are somehow "less than" their friends. They feel somehow inadequate.

The best thing you can do alleviate guilt and shame is to take control. You can't do anything about having asthma, but you can do something about how you treat it. Those who learn about asthma and follow their treatment plans often need less medicine, have fewer doctor's visits, and miss less time from school. They have fewer episodes and their day-to-day breathing is better. Today, there are newer once-a-day medications that can provide relief without having to rely as much on rescue inhalers. If using your inhaler in front of others is a problem for you, talk to your doctor about less visible treatment plans.

MY TEACHERS DON'T UNDERSTAND

Young people said teachers and coaches often don't know enough about asthma. They either underestimate the severity of the problem or they overreact.

Others said teachers sometimes compare them with other students who have asthma. Not realizing each teen with asthma is different, a teacher might not understand when one student can make it to school despite asthma and another with a more serious problem misses school. Coaches and gym teachers can underestimate the severity of the problem, some young people said. "They just think you are out of shape or lazy," one young woman told me. In her school, it was mandatory that each student run the mile in order to receive a fitness certificate.

"I would cry because I knew I was going to have to do it. It wasn't that I didn't want to do it; it was because I couldn't do it," she said. "I was fit. I just couldn't run that mile."

Many school systems now offer educational programs to help teachers and coaches understand asthma. If your school doesn't and your teachers or coaches don't seem to understand, ask your school nurse to talk to them for you. You will be helping yourself and other students the teachers see and you will help the adults become better informed.

RELIEF

Many teenagers actually feel relieved when they learn they have asthma. There is an explanation for the way they feel and there are treatments available to help them do the things they love to do. Seattle Seahawks linebacker Chad Brown had that type of reaction when he learned he had asthma. During his first year with the Seahawks, he found he couldn't play with the intensity he was used to. He couldn't play as hard because he couldn't breathe. In an interview with the Asthma Education Network, he said, ". . . being diagnosed with asthma was fantastic for me because I finally had an answer to what had been plaguing me. I approached it as a positive thing because now I knew what was going on and I knew there were treatments available." Gillian, a young woman who will join Brown University's rowing team this year, said something similar. She says treating her asthma is now "a way of life," not a huge obstacle. "It was harder when I did not know I had it. It was bad every night. I would wheeze and cough—that was annoying!"

YOU ARE NOT ALONE

No matter how you feel about asthma, you are not alone. When you consider that 14 million people have asthma, you can be sure that there are others out there feeling the same way you do. Some people with asthma have actually made themselves feel better by educating others. When you join a support group and share your feelings and information with others, it not only makes you feel better, but it helps the others in the group as well. Some young people like Amit Bushan in chapter 4 have become activists promoting healthy living. Young people like you have entered poster contests, gone on asthma walks, and created Web sites all designed to help others with asthma. Some find that relaxation techniques, like yoga and breathing exercises, help reduce worry and stress.

The best thing you can do for yourself is get on with your life. With the proper education and treatment, you can do the things you love to do. As they say at the "Teens and Asthma" page of the American Lung Association, "If you take your asthma seriously, you can get on with the serious business of having fun the rest of your life."

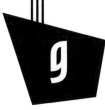

On Your Own

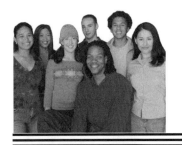

If you are a teenager with asthma, it won't be long before you are living independently. You will be graduating from high school and heading off to a college dorm or perhaps living with friends in an apartment and starting a new job. Once you have graduated from high school, your parents probably won't be supervising your health care. The desire to "do it myself" will become a reality. There is much excitement about leaving home and taking responsibility for yourself. If you have asthma, you need to take that into consideration when making plans for living independently. Much of the health-care running around your parents did for you will now be your job.

PREPLANNING

Before heading off on your own, get a check up. You should visit your doctor and tweak your action plan before you set out on your own. Be sure you know what medicines you will take routinely and what you should take if your asthma gets worse. Ask your doctor to give you a list of the medicines and keep the list with your prescription medicines. It will be handy should

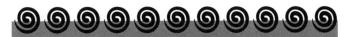

ASTHMA SCHOLARSHIPS

Did you know that there are college scholarships and grants available for young people with asthma? Students who play sports and also have asthma may be eligible for Schering/KEY's "The Will to Win Asthma Athlete Scholarships." If you are a student-athlete, in good academic standing, a U.S. citizen, and have been accepted to a bachelor's degree program at an accredited college, you could win a scholarship. For more information, call The Will to Win Scholarships Hotline at 1-800-558-7305.

The American Academy of Asthma, Allergy and Immunology, with the support of Aventis Pharmaceuticals, also sponsors a scholarship program for young people with asthma. Students need recommendations from a high-school principal or counselor and a verification of their condition from their allergist/immunologist or physician. A short essay is also required. Applications are available at the American Academy of Asthma, Allergy and Immunology home page at www.aaaai.org. Search *scholarship application* to learn more about the program.

Other programs may be available in your area. Ask your high-school guidance counselor for more information.

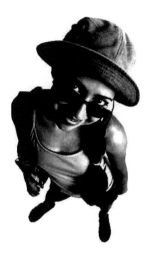

you need to visit the school health center or an emergency room. Be sure you have a toll-free number to get refills. Ask your at-home pharmacist how to go about this. If you have a mail prescription plan, call ahead to arrange to have refills delivered to you at school.

Ask for step-up or emergency prescriptions as well. You may need a round of nebulizer solutions or oral steroids if your asthma symptoms get bad. If you have a written prescription for those on hand, you can get your treatment underway and avoid an emergency room visit. Keep these written prescriptions with the other medicines so you will know where they are if you need them.

During your check-up, discuss drug and alcohol interactions. You should know that some asthma medicines can't be taken with some antibiotics. Some asthma medicines may cause a reaction if you drink alcohol. Don't be embarrassed to talk to your doctor about these interactions. It is better to be safe than to end up in an emergency room.

REQUEST A COPY OF YOUR RECORDS TO TAKE WITH YOU TO SCHOOL

If you are taking allergy shots, arrange to continue your shots while you are away. The doctor should be able to transfer the serum and instructions to the student health center.

Ask your doctor for several business cards and take them with you when you go to school. Put them in your medicine case and you will have them on hand if you need to visit the student health center or the emergency room.

If you are going to be far from home and your doctor, ask your doctor to recommend an asthma specialist near your school. You will need to arrange to have copies of your medical records, your management plan, and your insurance and prescription information sent to the doctor's office, and it would be wise to schedule an introductory appointment with the doctor before you leave home.

If you don't already have a spacer to use with your inhaled medicines, consider adding one now.

HEALTH INSURANCE

If you are covered by your parents' health plan, find out if you will be covered while you are at college. If not or if you don't have insurance, most schools offer insurance plans for students. There are fees for these health plans and all are different. Some cover pre-existing conditions like asthma and some don't. Ask if your college offers a plan and exactly what it will cover.

MEDICINE CHEST

Keep your medicines in a dry place. A plastic tub with a lid makes a good storage container for your medicines. Tape a list of your medicines and dosages to the lid of the case. Put your insurance information there as well. Keep a separate rescue case. Put your rescue inhaler and EpiPen (if you use one) in a separate container and carry them with you. Almost no one leaves a dorm without a backpack these days. Put your rescue kit in your backpack and take it with you wherever you go.

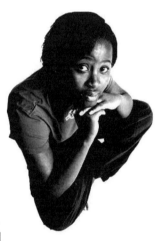

PEAK FLOW

If you don't already use a peak flow monitor, consider using one now. Communal living presents opportunities to be exposed to a variety of asthma triggers. Smoke, mildew, cold germs, viruses, perfumes, colognes, and spray deodorants will be a part of your life. Although you can do your best to avoid them, you will be exposed to more irritants than when you were living at home. If you use a peak flow meter and keep a record of your readings, you will know if there is trouble ahead before symptoms get out of control. You will be able to make adjustments to your treatment plan as needed.

HOUSING AND HOUSEKEEPING

If you are heading off to college or going to share an apartment, one of the most important decisions will be to

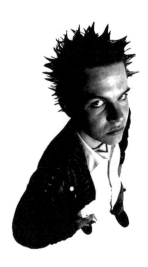

make your new home a no-smoking environment. If you will be living with friends, that needs to be understood upfront before signing any rental agreements. Your roommates will need to agree to the no-smoking policy and all of you will need to let visitors know that smoking is not allowed in what will be your home. If you are allergic to animals, you need to agree to a no-pets policy as well.

For those heading off to college, be sure you select a non-smoking dorm. Simply requesting a non-smoking roommate isn't enough. Dorms are usually congested. Hallways, bathrooms, and common rooms are shared. If smoking is allowed anywhere in the building, the smoke will reach you. At some colleges, all dorm rooms are non-smoking. Be sure to ask when visiting the college campus.

The bathroom can present additional problems. Mold and mildew can grow there. If there is mold in the bathroom, exchange jobs with your roommate. Have him or her clean the bathroom while you do a non-trigger task.

Roommates who use scented spray deodorants, hair spray, and/or perfume can create airborne irritants without even realizing it. Ask your roommates not to use these products, or at the very least, to use unscented varieties. Have them run the exhaust fan in the bathroom if they insist on using products that are triggers for you.

DECORATING

It is not unusual for first apartments or dorm rooms to be messy. Often students on their own for the first time take pleasure in making messes that weren't tolerated at home. Although this might seem like fun, if you have asthma, you are asking for trouble. You need to take the same care away from home as you did at home. Mite-proof pillow and mattress covers will help prevent asthma episodes. You will need to do laundry more often than your roommates. Wash your sheets and blankets to get rid of dust mites once a week. If your dorm has bunks, ask for the top bunk. That way the dust and allergens from the upper bunk won't drop down on you

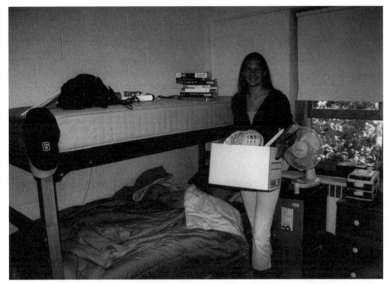

Katie in dorm room

Photo: Penny Paquette

Dorm rooms need special consideration. Katie has a simple window treatment on her window and has chosen the top bunk. She may decide to put special covers on her mattress and pillow. Her dorm room floor is bare.

as you sleep. You should consider running a HEPA room air filter to help reduce allergens in your room or apartment.

Keep floors bare and window treatments simple. Carpets and curtains gather dust.

SOCIAL SITUATIONS

Tell your roommate and your dorm adviser that you have asthma. Explain that you know how to control your symptoms, but that asthma episodes occasionally occur suddenly. Let them know what they should do if you have a problem.

One of the most difficult social problems on college campuses comes not from young people, but from cigarette smoke. Several young people I talked to said they had trouble with cigarette smoke in restaurants and bars. It is difficult for them to meet friends in areas where smoking is allowed. Unfortunately, that probably includes many social gathering areas on and around college campuses. Many fraternities allow smoking in their houses, but smoking isn't allowed in most public areas on college campuses. Most restaurants and fast-food establishments have no-smoking areas now. Choose one as your gathering place.

VACCINES

Many doctors suggest students with asthma have a flu vaccine. You will probably already be at school before flu vaccine season. Most colleges make the flu vaccine available to students. Ask your doctor if you should have a flu shot.

HEALTH CARE

Find out where the student health center is located and where to find the closest hospital. Visit the health center, introduce yourself, and give them a copy of your medical records and your action plan. Almost everyone gets sick during their first semester away from home. If your asthma symptoms get worse while you are at school, you will know where to go for help, and they will have a copy of your action plan to help treat you.

FOOD SERVICE

If you have food allergies be sure to arrange a meeting with the head of food services. They should be able to accommodate your food needs. Be sure they know about the risk of cross contamination of foods and that food allergies can be life threatening.

SUPPORT GROUPS

If you think you would like to join an asthma support group near your school, visit the student health center and ask about groups in the area. You can also contact the Asthma and Allergy Foundation for a group in the area. (See page 125 and the resources section at the end of the book.)

GENERAL HEALTH CARE

Wash your hands. Virus and bacterial infections are
common on college campuses and one of the things you can
do to avoid getting every bug that comes along is wash
your hands. Try to eat well, get enough rest, exercise, make
new friends, and have a great time.

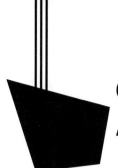

Glossary of Asthma Terms

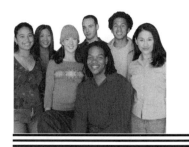

Action plan—A written plan developed by your doctor that outlines how to treat your asthma, when to increase medications, when to see the doctor, and when to seek emergency help. Also called an asthma management plan.

Acute—Brief (days to weeks).

Airways—A common term for the breathing tubes or bronchial tubes that move air into and out of your lungs.

Allergen—A substance that causes an allergic reaction in sensitive individuals such as certain foods, dust mites, animal dander, cockroaches, weeds, grass and tree pollens, mold and mildew, stinging insects, some drugs, some foods, certain dyes, cosmetics, and latex.

Allergic asthma—Reversible airway inflammation and obstruction triggered by an allergic reaction. See extrinsic asthma.

Allergic rhinitis—Inflammation of the mucus membranes in the nose, throat, sinuses, and/or ear passages that happens when you inhale an allergen. This is sometimes called hay fever.

Allergist—A specialist that takes care of people with allergies.

Allergy—An overreaction of the body's immune system to a specific allergen like dust or animal dander that cause allergy symptoms.

Alveoli—Millions of tiny air sacs in the lungs at the end of the airways that fill with air, allowing the gas exchange where blood picks up oxygen from the air breathed in and releases carbon dioxide to be exhaled.

Anaphylaxis—A severe, life-threatening allergic response. The reaction can occur after an insect sting or eating certain foods, or in reaction to an injected drug.

Animal dander—The invisible and sticky scales from an animal's skin that can cause an allergic reaction.

Antihistamines—Medicines that block the effects of histamines, the chemical that causes an allergic reaction.

Anti-inflammatory drugs—Medicines that reduce the symptoms and signs of inflammation.

Asthma—A chronic lung disease characterized by inflammation of the airways. Those with asthma have hypersensitive airways that overreact to irritants. Symptoms can include coughing, wheezing, shortness of breath, chest tightness, or excessive mucus production.

Asthma attack—When asthma symptoms get worse or intensify and breathing becomes difficult. Sometimes called an asthma episode or an exacerbation.

Asthma management plan—See action plan.

Atopic dermatitis—See Eczema.

Atopy—The tendency to develop an allergy.

Beta agonist—Also called a beta-2 agonist, it is the most common type of bronchodilator medicine. The medicine enhances the stimulation of the beta-2 type automatic nerve that is responsible for relaxing the airway muscles and opening the airways.

Bronchi—The airways that lead from the trachea to each lung, subdivide into smaller and smaller branches, then connect with the bronchioles.

Bronchial tubes—The tubes that let air into and out of the lungs.

Bronchiole—The tiny airways that branch from the bronchi to the alveoli.

Bronchitis—An infection or inflammation in the bronchial tubes.

Bronchodilator—Medicines that relax the smooth muscles of the airways allowing them to open up.

Bronchospasm—The tightening of the muscles of the airways.

Chronic—Ongoing or continuing. Remaining for several years or for a lifetime.

Controller medicines—Drugs (oral and inhaled) that are used on a long-term basis to get asthma symptoms under control. They can include anti-inflammatory agents and long-acting bronchodilators. Sometimes called preventer or prophylactic medicines.

Corticosteroids—A medication that reduces airway swelling, making it easier to breathe.

Eczema—An inflammation of the skin, usually causing itching and sometimes crusting, scaling, or blisters on the skin. When the skin condition is made worse by allergic factors, it is called atopic dermatitis.

Epinephrine—A naturally occurring hormone, also called adrenaline, that increases the speed and force of heart beats. It opens the airways to improve breathing and narrows blood vessels in the skin and intestines so that more blood reaches the muscles.

EpiPen—The brand name of a device used to deliver epinephrine, a medicine used for quick relief during life-threatening medical emergencies.

Exacerbate—To make worse.

Exacerbation—Any worsening of symptoms, whether acute or gradual. See asthma attack.

Exercise-induced asthma—Asthma symptoms that begin during or following exercise. Symptoms can be minor or severe.

Extrinsic asthma—Asthma that is triggered by an allergic reaction, usually something inhaled or in the environment. See allergic asthma.

Gastroesophageal reflux disease (GERD)—A disorder in which some of the acid and enzymes from the stomach flow up into the esophagus, leading to what is commonly called heartburn. It is more common in people with asthma and is a trigger for some.

Histamine—A chemical in cells throughout the body that is released during an allergic or inflammatory reaction. It can cause the narrowing of the airways during an asthma attack.

Hives—See Urticaria.

Hyperresponsiveness—The hyperactivity of the airways, sometimes called twitchiness, that is a symptom of asthma.

Immune system—The collection of cells and proteins that protects the body from potentially harmful, infectious microorganisms such as bacteria, viruses and fungi.

Immunoglobulin E (IgE)—A type of antibody formed to protect the body from infection that attaches to mast cells in the respiratory and intestinal tracts and may cause allergic rhinitis, asthma, or eczema. These antibodies are normally present in very low levels, but are found in larger numbers in people with allergies.

Immunoglobulins—Also known as antibodies, they bind to substances in the body that are recognized as foreign antigens. This binding helps destroy the microorganisms that bear the antigens. They play an important role in allergies when they bind to antigens that are not necessarily a threat and cause inflammation.

Immunotherapy—Injections that help prevent and reduce inflammation in both allergic rhinitis and allergic asthma.

Inhaler—See metered-dose inhaler.

Intrinsic asthma—Asthma with no apparent external cause—non-allergic.

Intubation—The process of putting a tube down someone's throat into the trachea. The tube is connected to a machine that pushes measured amounts of air into the lungs and then lets it out to help a person breathe.

Irritant—A trigger that can cause increased symptoms.

Leukotriene—A chemical involved in inflammation that seem to play an important role in the inflammation associated with asthma. Newer asthma medicines called antileukotrienes help to reduce leukotrienes or limit their effects.

Leukotriene modifiers—Medicines used to reduce inflammation by reducing a chemical called leukotriene.

Lung function—A measure of how well the lungs are working.

Lymphocyte—Any group of white blood cells that are an essential part of the immune system and carry out a very specific defense against dangerous invading organisms that penetrate the body's more general defenses.

Mast cell—Cells that play an important role in the body's allergic response. Commonly found on the surfaces of the nose, throat, and bronchial tubes, they release chemicals that cause redness and swelling during an allergic reaction.

Metered-dose inhaler (MDI)—A delivery system for commonly prescribed asthma medications that delivers the medicine in a premeasured dose when you inhale. Sometimes called a puffer.

Mucus—The fluid that coats and protects the inside of the nose, mouth, bronchial tubes, and other parts of the body. Those with asthma sometimes produce excessive mucus that clogs the narrowed airways.

Nebulizer—A machine that turns asthma medicine into mist allowing it to be inhaled.

Peak flow—A measure of the fastest speed at which you can blow air out of your lungs.

Peak flow meter—A small device that measures how fast you can blow air out of your lungs.

Preventer medicines—Drugs that are taken over a long period of time to reduce the number and severity of asthma attacks. Sometimes called controller medicines.

Puff—A term used to indicate how many times you should inhale (or puff) medicine from a metered-dose inhaler.

Puffer—See metered-dose inhaler.

RAST—RadioAllergoSorbent Test is a trademarked test used to detect IgE antibodies in specific allergens.

Reliever medicine—Sometimes called rescue medicine or quick-relief medicine. These medicines act quickly to help reverse asthma symptoms such as airway swelling, wheezing, and coughing.

Rhinitis—See allergic rhinitis.

Sinus—The air cavities within the facial bones that are lined with mucus membranes similar to those in other airways.

Sinusitis—An inflammation in the sinus cavities, often caused by bacterial or viral infections.

Spacer—A device, sometimes called an aerochamber, that attaches to an inhaler to help deliver the medicine more efficiently.

Spasm—A sudden, strong muscle tightening.

Spirometer—A machine used to measure the air that moves in and out of the lungs.

Systemic—Affecting the body as a whole rather than one specific area or organ.

Theophylline—A bronchodilator drug that widens the airways to the lung.

Trachea—The largest breathing tube in the body that passes from the throat down to the chest.

Trigger—Something that makes asthma symptoms appear or worsen.

Upper respiratory system—The parts of the body used for breathing: nose, throat, airways.

Urticaria—A skin condition commonly known as hives.

Wheeze—The whistling sound often associated with asthma. It is created when air moves through the narrowed airways.

Zone—An area in the asthma action plan that helps define and monitor the severity of asthma symptoms.

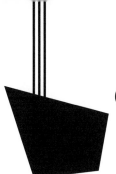

Chapter Notes

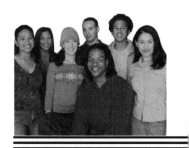

CHAPTER 1

Arab, Sameh M. "Medicine in Ancient Egypt." www. arabworldbooks.com/articles8.htm (2 April 2002).

Ashworth, Allan. "Cardano's Solution (Girolamo Cardano's Works)." *History Today*, January 1999.

"Asthma Through the Ages." Merck & Company, Inc. www.merck.com/disease/asthma/asthma_timeline/home2.ht ml (4 April 2002).

"Asthma Through the Ages." Asthmaline.com. www.asthmaline. com/HIST/HIST02.htm (1 April 2002).

Bloch, Sydney. "Moses Maimonides' Contribution to the Biopsychosocial Approach in Clinical Medicine." *Lancet*, 8 September 2002.

"Breath of Life." National Library of Medicine. www.nlm.nih. gov/hmd/breath/breathhome.html (4 April 2002).

Salter, H. H. *On Asthma: Its Pathology and Treatment*. 2nd ed. London, England: Churchill, 1898.

Woodcock, Ashley. "Allergen Avoidance." State of the art lecture at the annual meeting of the Swiss Society of Pneumology (Lausanne, 15–16 June 2000). www.smw.ch/pdf/2000_49/ 2000-49-246.pdf (5 April 2002).

CHAPTER 2

"Anatomy Lesson—Asthma 101." Asthma and Allergy Network /Mothers of Asthmatics. www.aanma.org/schoolhouse/sh_ anatomylesson.htm (5 June 2002).

"Asthma Basics." National Institute of Allergy and Infectious Diseases, National Institutes of Health. www.niaid.nih.gov/ newsroom/focuson/asthma01/basics Htm (18 April 2002).

"Breath of Life: Faces of Asthma." National Library of Medicine, National Institutes of Health. www.nlm.nih.gov/hmd/breath/ Faces_asthma/facesframe.html (10 July 2002).

"Fast Facts: Famous People with Asthma." American Academy of Allergy, Asthma, and Immunology. www.aaaai.org/public/fastfacts/famous.stm (11 October 2001).

Hannaway, Paul. *Asthma: The Emerging Epidemic*. Marblehead, Mass.: Lighthouse Press, 2002.

CHAPTER 3

"All About Atopic Dermatitis." National Eczema Association, 1999. www.nationaleczama.org/lwe/allabout_atopic_dermatitis.html (6 June 2002).

"Asthmatics Can Excel in Sports." American Academy of Allergy, Asthma and Immunology, 16 January 2002. www.aaaai.org/media/news_releases/2002/01/011602.html (2 June 2002).

"Atopic Dermatitis in Children." National Eczema Association, 1998. www.nationaleczema.org/lwe/atopic_dermatitis_children.html (6 July 2002).

Babu, K. Suresh, and Sundeep S. Salvi. "Aspirin and Asthma." American College of Chest Physicians, *Chest* 2000.

"Black Asthmatics More Resistant to Steroids: Study." Yale New Haven Health, Reuters Health, May 2002. yalenewhavenhealth.org/healthnews/reuters/NewsStory0527200221.htm (7 June 2002).

"Black Teenagers with Severe Asthma are Three Times More Likely Than White Teens to Have Steroid-Resistant Asthma." National Jewish Medical and Research Center, 23 July 1998. nationaljewish.org/news/98july23.html (2 July 2002).

Blaiss, Michael S. "Researchers Urge Identification and Treatment of Comorbid Conditions Related to Asthma." Conference Coverage, 58th Annual Meeting of the American Academy of Allergy, Asthma and Immunology, 12 April 2002. www.medscape.com (15 April 2002).

"Bronchiectasis." Canadian Lung Association, May 22, 2002. www.lung.ca/diseases/bronchiectasis.html (27 June 2002).

"Emphysema and Chronic Bronchitis: What is COPD?" National Jewish Medical and Research Center, 12 June 2002. nationaljewish.org/understanding/emphysemachronicbronchitis.html (26 February 2002).

"Emphysema Bytes." National Jewish Medical and Research Center, 12 June 2002. nationaljewish.org/emphysemabytes.html (27 June 2002).

Essential Guide to Asthma. American Medical Association. New York: Simon and Schuster, 1998.

"Facts About Cystic Fibrosis." National Institutes of Health, National Health Lung and Blood Institute. NIH Publication No. 95-3650, November 1995.

"Global Initiative for Asthma." National Institutes of Health, National Heart, Lung, and Blood Institute, 2002. www. ginasthma.com/pocketguide/pocket.html (8 April 2002).

"Guidelines for the Diagnosis and Management of Asthma— Update on Selected Topics 2002." NIH Publication No. 02-5075, June 2002.

"Just for Kids: Letter from Kurt Grote." American Academy of Allergy, Asthma and Immunology. www.aaaai.org/patients/ just4kids/grote/letter.stm (3 April 2002).

Medicine in Quotations Online. www.acponline.org/cgi-bin/ medquotes.pl.

"Occupational Asthma." Occupational Safety and Health Administration, U.S. Department of Labor. www.osha-slc. gov/oshinfo/priorities/asthma.html (15 April 2002).

Papazian, Ruth. "On the Teen Scene: Being a Sport with Exercise-Induced Asthma." *FDA Consumer Magazine*, January–February 1994. www.fda.gov/fdac/reprints/ots_asth.html (2 June 2002).

"A Pocket Guide for Physicians and Nurses." National Institutes of Health, National Heart, Lung, and Blood Institute, 1998.

"Practical Guide for the Diagnosis and Management of Asthma." U.S. Department of Health and Human Services, National Institutes of Health, National Heart, Lung, and Blood Institute. NIH No. 97-4053, October 1997.

Siette, Gregory B., et al. "Nocturnal Asthma in Children Affects School Attendance, School Performance, and Parents' Work Attendance." *Archives of Pediatrics and Adolescent Medicine*, September 2000. archpedi.ama-assn.org (15 April 2002).

"Steroid-Resistant Asthma." Harvard Medical School Consumer Health Information, InteliHealth, 18 February 2002. www.intelihealth.com/IH/ihtIH/WSIHW000/3457/6923/258 876.html?d=dmtContent (10 April 2002).

"Tips to Remember: Exercise-Induced Asthma." American Academy of Allergy, Asthma and Immunology. www.aaaai. org/patients/publicedmat/tips/exerciseinducedasthma.stm (2 July 2002).

Weersink, E. J. M., et al. "Controlling Nighttime Asthma May Improve Daytime Cognitive Performance in Asthmatics." *American Journal of Respiratory and Critical Care Medicine*, 16 October 1997. www.lungusa.org/press/asthmamedcontrol.html (15 April 2002).

"What is CF?" Cystic Fibrosis Foundation. www.cff.org/about_cf/what_is_cf.cfm/CFID=8967&CFTOKEN=51537322 (27 June 2002).

CHAPTER 4

"A Brief Guide to Mold, Moisture, and Your Home." U.S. Environmental Protection Agency, 22 April 2002. www.epa.gov/iag/molds/moldguide.html (27 May 2002).

"Asthma Triggers—Related Topics—Combustion Pollutants." U.S. Environmental Protection Agency, 8 April 2002. www.epa.gov.iaq/asthma/triggers/combust.html (19 May 2002).

"Cockroach Control Guide." Environmental Health Watch, 22 April 2002. www.ehw.org/Asthma/ASTH_Cockroach_Control.htm (6 May 2002).

Cook, Gretchen. "When Weather Worsens Asthma: A Storm of Asthma Triggers May be Blowing Your Way." *Asthma Magazine*, July/August 2001.

"Essential Guide to Asthma." American Medical Association. New York: Pocket Books, 1998.

Formanek, Raymond. "Food Allergies: When Food Becomes the Enemy." *FDA Consumer Magazine*, July/August 2001.

"Get Rid of Whom?" Allergy and Asthma Network/Mothers of Asthmatics. www.aanma.org/homesweet/hs_getridofwho.htm (17 July 2002).

"Guidelines on Assessment and Remediation of Fungi in Indoor Environments." New York City Department of Health, Bureau of Environmental and Occupational Disease Epidemiology. www.ci.nyc.ny.us/html/doh/html/epi/moldrpt1.html (7 May 2002).

"Health Precautions During Mold Cleanup and Removal." North Carolina Department of Health and Human Services. www.epi.state.nc.us/epi/oii/mold/precautions.html (7 May 2002).

"Heroin Inhalation May Trigger Life-Threatening Asthma," *Pulmonary Reviews*, June 2000.

"Home Sweet Home: Battling Mold." Allergy and Asthma
  Network/Mothers of Asthmatics. www.aanma.org/
  homesweet/hs_battlingmold.htm (17 July 2002).

"How to Create a Dust-Free Bedroom." National Institute of
  Allergy and Infectious Disease. October 2001.
  www.niaid.nih.gov/factsheets/dustfree.htm (17 July 2002).

Mallozzi, Vincent M. "A Nation Challenged: Charity; For
  Asthmatic Children, An Extra Health Burden." *New York
  Times,* 20 September 2001.

Maremont, Mark, and Jared Sandberg. "Tests Say Air is Safe, But
  Some People Feel Ill near Ground Zero." *Wall Street
  Journal,* 26 December 2002.

Matthews, Karen. "Effects of Terror Attack on Children Not
  Known." Associated Press. C-Health. www.canoe.ca/
  Health0202/21_terror-ap.html (19 July 2002).

"Mold Allergy." National Institute of Allergy and Infectious
  Diseases, National Institutes of Health, 4 April 2001.
  www.niaid.hih.gov/publications/allergens/mold.htm
  (22 February 2002).

"Monosodium Glutamate." Food and Drug Administration,
  31 August 1995. www.fda/gov/opacom/backgrounders/
  msg.html (21 May 2002).

Moss, Abigail J., et al. "Recent Trends in Adolescent Smoking,
  Smoking-Uptake Correlates, and Expectations About the
  Future." Advance Data No. 221. U.S. Department of Health
  and Human Services, Centers for Disease Control and
  Prevention, 2 December 1992.

Musto, Pat. "Pollution and Asthma." *Allergy and Asthma
  Advocate*, Fall 2001. www.aaaai.org/patients/advocate/
  2001/fall/pollution.stm. (17 May 2002).

"NIAID Study: Cockroaches Important Cause of Asthma
  Morbidity Among Inner-City Children." National Institute
  of Allergy and Infectious Disease, 7 May 1997.
  www.niaid.nih.gov/newsroom/releases/asthmanr.htm 5/7/02.

Papazian, Ruth. "Sulfites: Safe for Most, Dangerous for Some."
  FDA Consumer Magazine, December 1996.
  www.fda/gpv/fdac/features/096_suf.html. (21 May 2002).

"Power Plants Linked to Asthma." *USA Today,* 5 May 2000.
  www.usatoday.com/life/health/allergies/lhall011.htm
  (7 June 2002).

Sandler, Nancy. *A Parents Guide to Asthma.* New York:
  Doubleday, 1989.

"The State of the Air 2002 Report." The American Lung Association, 2002. www.lungusa.org/air2001/index.html (22 February 2002).

"Threat From Mouse Allergens" Johns Hopkins Medical Institutions, Health Newsfeed #1457. www.hopkinsmedicine. org/healthnewsfeed/hnf_1457.htm (7 May 2002).

"Tobacco Use Among Middle and High School Students— National Youth Tobacco Survey 1999." Centers for Disease Control. www.cdc.gov/tobacco/research_data/survey/ mmwr4903fs.htm (1 May 2002).

Watson, Traci. "Fires' Dangers Drift Far Beyond Flames." *USA Today*, 8 July 2002. www.usatoday.com/news/nation/ 2002/07/09/fire-danger.htm (16 July 2002).

"What is Reye's Syndrome?" National Reye's Syndrome Foundation, Inc. www.reyessyndrome.org/what.htm (30 August 2002).

Whole Truth Website. Florida Department of Health. www.wholetruth.com (2 May 2002).

Wood, Robert A. "The Real Truth About Cats and Dogs." Asthma and Allergy Network/Mothers of Asthmatics. www.aanma.org/petshop/ps_truth.htm (6 May 2002).

CHAPTER 5

"Anti-IgE Treatment: What is Anti-IgE Treatment?" National Jewish Medical and Research Center, 2000. www.njc.org/ medfacts/anti_ige.html (26 March 2002).

"April Medical Release: Studies Find Many Teens with Asthma Lack Basic Knowledge About Controlling Their Disease." American Lung Association, 15 April 1999. www.lungusa. org/press/medical/medapril99_two.html (17 April 2002).

"Controlling Your Asthma." National Institutes of Health. September 1997.

"Corticosteroids vs. Anabolic Steroids." Glaxo Wellcome, Inc., Memorial Care Asthma Newsletter CMD295RO, January 1999. www.memorialcare.com/stories/steroids.cfm (30 February 2002).

"Defective Gene Holds Asthma Clue." Health eHeadlines, 10 July 2002. American Academy of Allergy, Asthma and Immunology. www.aaaai.org/news/SITEWare/output/ html/2002/07/10/eng-pressassociation_health_long/eng-pressassociation_health_long_034301_11_1456454102881. stm (11 July 2002).

"Five Asthma Medication Groups." American Lung Association, March 2002. www.lungusa.org/asthma/ascastnedgr.html (15 April 2002).

Flieger, Ken. "Controlling Asthma." U.S. Food and Drug Administration, June 2000. www.fda.gov/fdac/features/ 966_asth.html (21 February 2002).

"Forest Fires in West Could Mean Health Problems for Asthmatics." American Academy of Allergy, Asthma and Immunology, June 2002. www.aaaai.org/media/news_ releases/2002/06/062702.html (5 July 2002).

"Global Strategy for Asthma Management and Prevention (GINA Report)." National Institutes of Health, National Heart, Lung, and Blood Institute, 2002.

"Guidelines for the Diagnosis and Management of Asthma— Update on Selected Topics 2002." NIH Publication No. 02-5075. National Institutes of Health, National Heart, Lung, and Blood Institute.

Hannaway, Paul J. "Asthma and Allergy Alert: Immunotherapy." Marblehead: Lighthouse Press and Allergy and Asthma Affiliates of the North Shore, 2002.

Moran, W. Reed. "Jerome Bettis Shares Asthma Game Plan." USA Today, 2 September 2001. www.usatoday.com/news/ health/spotlight/2001-09-04-bettis-asthma.htm (1 April 2002).

"NHLBI Supported Study Finds Inhaled Steroids Accelerate Bone Loss in Women with Asthma." NIH News Release, National Heart, Lung, and Blood Institute, 26 September 2001. www.nhlbi.nih.gov/new/press/01/09/26.htm (31 May 2002).

"Prescription Medication Assistance Programs." Allergy and Asthma/Mothers of Asthmatics. www.aanma.org/pharmacy/ ph_medassist.htm (29 May 2002).

Stemple, David A. "Growth and Inhaled Corticosteroids: Answers for Your Patients." Medscape Conference Coverage, 12 April 2002. www.medscape.com/viewarticle/431526 (31 May 2002).

"Treating Bacterial Infections Can Help Asthmatics." National Jewish Medical and Research Center, 11 June 2002. www.njc.org/news/clari_asthma.html (25 June 2002).

"Trends in Allergic Disease." Media Resources Kit, American Academy of Allergy, Asthma and Immunology. www.aaaai.org/media/resources/media_kit/trends_in_allergic_disease.stm (18 April 2002).

"Update on National Asthma Guidelines Release." NIH News Release, National Institutes of Health, National Heart, Lung, and Blood Institute, 10 June 2002. www.nhlbi.nih.gov/new/press/02-06-10.htm (1 July 2002).

"Use of Steroids for Asthma and Allergies (Tip #6)." American Academy of Allergy, Asthma and Immunology: Milwaukee, Wisconsin, 1995.

"Using an Action Plan to Manage Your Asthma: Medfacts." National Jewish Medical and Research Center, 22 May 2002. www.njc.org/medfacts/asthma_action_plan.html (24 May 2002).

"Your Metered-Dose Inhaler Will be Changing . . . Here are the Facts." National Heart, Lung, and Blood Institute. www.nhlbi.nih.gov/health/public/lung/asthma/mdi.htm (27 May 2002).

CHAPTER 6

"Asthma and Physical Activity in School." National Heart, Lung, and Blood Institute, National Institutes of Health, September 1995. www.nhlbi.nih.gov/health/public/lung/asthma/phy_astr.htm#ensure (13 June 2002).

"Children's Rights at School." Allergy and Asthma Network, Mothers of Asthmatics (AANMA). www.aanma.org/cityhall/ch_childrights.htm (16 September 2002).

Childs, Michael. "UGA Education Researchers Say Study Suggests Teachers Should be Trained to Manage Students with Asthma." The University of Georgia News Bureau, 29 January 2002. www.uga.edu/news/newsbureau/releases/2002releases/0201020129asthma.html (20 June 2002).

"How Asthma-Friendly is Your School?" *Journal of the American Medical Association*, 1999. www.ama-assn.org/special/asthma/newsline/special/how.htm (21 September 2001).

"National Asthma Education and Prevention Program (NAEPP): Resolution on Asthma Management at School." National Heart, Lung, and Blood Institute, National Institutes of Health. www.nhlbi.nih.gov/health/public/lung/asthma/resolut.htm (13 June 2002).

"National Survey of School Nurses Reveals the Challenge of Managing Asthma at School." *Asthma Magazine*, PR Newswire, 18 May 1999. calnurse.org/can/news/yah05199.html (20 June 2002).

"Nighttime Asthma Squeezes School Attendance." Johns Hopkins Medical Institutions, 25 April 1999. www.hopkinsmedicine.org/press/1999/APRIL99/990425.HTM (20 June 2002).

Weinberger, Miles. "Information for School Personnel Regarding Treatment of Asthma." Children's Hospital of Iowa, Virtual; Children's Hospital, 10 January 2000. www.vh.org/Patients/IHB/Peds/Allergy/Asthma/13School.html (20 June 2002).

"What Parents Need to Know About Diesel School Buses." Natural Resources Defense Council, 17 March 2002. www.nrdc.org/air/transportation/qbus.asp (2 October 2001).

"Why Indoor Air Quality is Important to your School." U.S. Environmental Protection Agency, 23 April 2002. www.epa.gov/iaq/schools/scholkit.html (25 May 2002).

CHAPTER 7

"Asthma: A Concern for Minority Populations." National Institutes of Health, National Institute of Allergy and Infectious Disease, October 2001. www.niaid.nih.gov/factsheets/asthma.htm (7 May 2002).

"Children's Risk of Death From Asthma Linked to Family Dysfunction." Doctor's Guide Global Edition, 19 May 1998. www.pslgroup.com/dg/7ce6a.htm (18 November 2001).

Gerland, Erwin W. "Fatal or Near-Fatal Asthma: A Continuing Threat." Conference Coverage: 58th Annual Meeting of the American Academy of Allergy, Asthma and Immunology. Medscape, 12 April 2002. www.medscape.com/viewarticle/431523 (15 April 2002).

"New Asthma Estimates: Tracking Prevalence, Heath Care, and Mortality." National Centers for Health Statistics, 5 October 2001. www.cdc.gov/nchs/products/pubs/pubd/hestats/asthma/asthma.htm (7 June 2002).

Randolph, Christopher. "Teen Asthma: A Complex Problem." American Academy of Allergy, Asthma and Immunology, August 2000. www.aaaai.org/members/academynews/2001/08/teenasthma.stm (20 May 2002).

CHAPTER 8

"Brief Writing Exercises Can Reduce Symptoms in Patients with Chronic Illness: Shown to be Effective for Asthma and Rheumatoid Arthritis." *Journal of the American Medical Association,* 4 April 1999. www.ama-assn.org/sci-pubs/sci-news/1999/snr0414.htm (9 July 2002).

"Chat Transcript: Olympic Swimmer Amy Van Dyken on Managing Asthma." CNN.com, 27 April 1999. www.cnn.com/HEALTH/9910/27/chat.vandyken (25 July 2002).

"Emotional and Social Effects." All About Asthma. University of Chicago Asthma Center. asthma.bsd.uchicago.edu/AboutAsthma/AAEmo.html (6 July 2002).

"Living with Asthma: One Day at a Time." ibreathe.com, GlaxoSmithKline. www.gsk.ibreathe.com (6 July 2002).

"Society and Self." Asthma Assistant Self-Management Web Site. www.asthmaassistant.com/tp2self/society.html (6 July 2002).

CHAPTER 9

"College Survival Guide, Allergy and Asthma." Network Mothers of America. www.aanma.org/schoolhouse/sh_collegesurvival.htm (7 July 2002).

Gonsior, Elaine C. "Asthma and the College Student." *Allergy and Asthma Advocate,* American Academy of Allergy, Asthma and Immunology, Summer 2000.

"Your College Student and Asthma." FreeBreather. www.asthmalerninglab.com (9 July 2002).

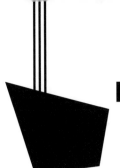

Resources

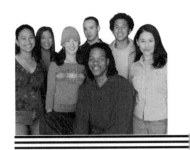

BOOK RESOURCES

Fiction

Bradley, Kimberly Brubaker. *Weaver's Daughter*. New York: Delacorte, 2000.
Each autumn brings chest pains and breathing problems for a 10-year-old pioneer girl living in the Southwest Territory in the 1790s. Lizzy knows she could die, but she chooses to live life as fully as possible. Includes information about early medical practices.
Getz David. *Thin Air*. New York: Henry Holt, 1990.
A funny story about a young man and his struggles to overcome his asthma and his overprotective brother.
Thesman, Jean. *Appointment with a Stranger*. New York: Avon, 1990.
High-school student Keller Parrish, who suffers severe asthma attacks, meets a mysterious young man at a remote pond, unaware that he is a ghost. This book may be out of print. Check your local library for a copy.

Non-Fiction

Adams, Francis V. *The Asthma Sourcebook, 2nd Edition*. Los Angeles: Lowell House, 1998.
American Medical Association. *Essential Guide to Asthma*. New York: Simon and Schuster, 1998.
Hannaway, Paul. *Asthma: An Emerging Epidemic*. Marblehead, Mass.: Lighthouse Press, 2002.

Organizations and Online Resources

American Academy of Allergy, Asthma and Immunology
611 East Wells Street
Milwaukee, WI 53202
1-800-822-2762
www.aaaai.org

American College of Allergy, Asthma and Immunology
85 West Algonquin Road
Suite 550
Arlington Heights, IL 60005
708-727-1200
allergy.mcg.edu

American Lung Association
Local Chapter
1-800-LUNG-USA
National Headquarters
1740 Broadway
New York, NY
212-315-8700
www.lungusa.org

Asthma and Allergy Foundation of America
1125 15th Street, NW
Suite 502
Washington, DC 20005
1-800-7-ASTHMA
www.aafa.org

Allergy and Asthma Network—Mothers of Asthmatics, Inc.
2751 Prosperity Avenue
Suite 150
Fairfax, VA 22031
1-800-878-4403
www.aanma.org

The Food Allergy and Anaphylaxis Network
10400 Eaton Place
Suite 107
Fairfax, VA 22030-12208
1-800-929-4040
www.foodallergy.org

National Asthma Education and Prevention Program
    301-251-1222
    www.nhlbi.nih.gov/health/public/lung/index.htm

National Institutes of Health
    Information Center
    P.O. Box 30105
    Bethesda, MD 20824-0105
    www.nhlbi.nih.gov

National Jewish Medical and Research Center
    1400 Jackson Street
    Denver, CO 80206
    303-388-4461
    www.NationalJewish.org

Lung Line
    1-800-222-LUNG
    Talk to a nurse and request printed information

National Institute of Allergy and Infectious Diseases
    NIAID Office of Communications
    www.niaid.nih.gov/publications

U.S. Environmental Protection Agency
    www.epa.gov/iaq

Support Groups

American Lung Association
    Lung Lounge Chat Room
    www.lungusa.org/chat

Asthma and Allergy Foundation of America
    Education Support Groups
    www.aafa.org/templ/display.cfm?id=44
    Click "ESG" search to find a group near you

Index

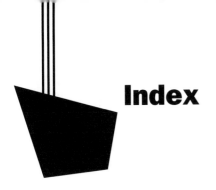

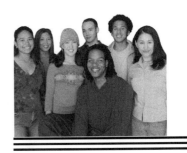

Italicized page numbers indicate photos.

Index

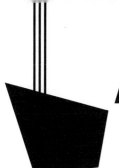

About the Author

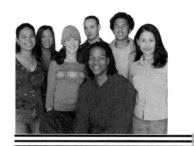

Penny Paquette is an educational writer and former school librarian. She has a wealth of experience helping teenagers find appropriate books to help them with their concerns. For this book, she brings not only her expertise as a writer, but her personal experience as an asthmatic as well.

This is her second book for Scarecrow Press's *It Happened to Me* series. She is also the author of *Learning Disabilities: The Ultimate Teen Guide.*

In addition to writing for teenagers, she is the coauthor of *Parenting a Child with a Learning Disability*, *Parenting a Child with a Behavior Problem*, and *Thinking Games to Play with Your Child.*